What Should We Do About Animal Welfare?

11/99.

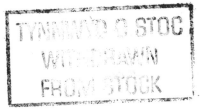

What Should We Do About Animal Welfare?

by Michael C. Appleby

Senior Lecturer in Farm Animal Behaviour
Institute of Ecology and Resource Management
University of Edinburgh

Blackwell
Science

© 1999 by
Blackwell Science Ltd
Editorial Offices:
Osney Mead, Oxford OX2 0EL
25 John Street, London WC1N 2BL
23 Ainslie Place, Edinburgh EH3 6AJ
350 Main Street, Malden
   MA 02148 5018, USA
54 University Street, Carlton
   Victoria 3053, Australia
10, rue Casimir Delavigne
   75006 Paris, France

Other Editorial Offices:

Blackwell Wissenschafts-Verlag GmbH
Kurfürstendamm 57
10707 Berlin, Germany

Blackwell Science KK
MG Kodenmacho Building
7-10 Kodenmacho Nihombashi
Chuo-ku, Tokyo 104, Japan

First published 1999

Set in 10.5/12.5pt Palatino
by DP Photosetting, Aylesbury, Bucks
Printed and bound in Great Britain by
MPG Books Ltd, Bodmin, Cornwall

The Blackwell Science logo is a trade
mark of Blackwell Science Ltd, registered
at the United Kingdom Trade Marks
Registry

DISTRIBUTORS

Marston Book Services Ltd
PO Box 269
Abingdon
Oxon OX14 4YN
(*Orders:* Tel: 01235 465500
           Fax: 01235 465555)

USA
Blackwell Science, Inc.
Commerce Place
350 Main Street
Malden, MA 02148 5018
(*Orders:* Tel: 800 759 6102
                 781 388 8250
           Fax: 781 388 8255)

Canada
Login Brothers Book Company
324 Saulteaux Crescent
Winnipeg, Manitoba R3J 3T2
(*Orders:* Tel: 204 837-2987
           Fax: 204 837-3116)

Australia
Blackwell Science Pty Ltd
54 University Street
Carlton, Victoria 3053
(*Orders:* Tel: 03 9347 0300
           Fax: 03 9347 5001)

A catalogue record for this title is
available from the British Library

ISBN 0–632–05066–7

Library of Congress
Cataloging-in-Publication Data
Appleby, Michael C.
    What should we do about animal
welfare? / by Michael C. Appleby.
        p.   cm.
    Includes bibliographical references
and index.
    ISBN 0-632-05066-7
    1. Animal welfare.   2. Human-
animal relationships.   I. Title.
HV4708.A66   1999
179'.3 – dc21   99-35003
                                 CIP

For further information on
Blackwell Science, visit our website:
www.blackwell-science.com

Contents

Preface

I have always been fascinated by animals. I did a zoology degree at university and then studied the behaviour of wild red deer in Scotland. After that I wanted to continue scientific work on animal behaviour, and also to address questions that were directly useful. That took me into research on farm animals. A major aspect of studying animal behaviour is the attempt to understand the animal's point of view. Why did that cow attack the farmer? Was she being aggressive or was she really frightened? Questions like that may start off as straightforward applied science (How can we protect the farmer?) but they rapidly raise the issue of animal welfare (How can we avoid the cow being frightened?). The shift was rapid, at least, in my own mind. Fascination is mingled with concern, and I went on to work on the understanding and improvement of animal welfare. Quite a lot of that work is mentioned in the book, but of course I also depend heavily on the research and writing of colleagues around the world.

The subject of animal welfare is constantly changing, and although it is difficult to hit a moving target I am glad to say that there are more positive changes than negative. While this book was at the proof stage there was a major, encouraging move forward in one area with which I am particularly involved: housing for laying hens (p. 118). It was not possible to change all references to battery cages at that stage, but then there will doubtless be other parts of the book that soon become out of date too. Let us hope so.

The need for a book like this has been evident to me for some time. The opportunity to make a start on planning and writing came with a Hume Fellowship from the Universities Federation for Animal Welfare which I was honoured to be awarded. UFAW funds research, information and education about welfare, and provides a welcome, moderate voice in an emotive field.

An important part of the planning was carried out in Copenhagen in discussions with Peter Sandøe, who considerably helped my understanding of ethics. While involved in the Fellowship I was also supported, as ever, by colleagues at the University of Edinburgh, and I am grateful both for that specific help and for general support of work on farm animal behaviour and welfare. It is, indeed, an indication of how attitudes are changing that my post – a lectureship in farm animal behaviour – was created at all, in what was then a university department of agriculture.

The following colleagues have generously and uncomplainingly read all the text and made many useful comments, and I am deeply indebted to them: Barry Hughes, Ute Knierim, Joy Mench, Anne Pankhurst, Peter Sandøe, Natalie Waran and Françoise Wemelsfelder. Thanks are due to Rachel Rodger for her attractive, original drawings. Lastly, I am sustained in all that I do by family and friends. I would like to dedicate this book to my brother John and to the memory of my brother Bob.

MCA

This book is dedicated to
John Appleby
and to the memory of
Robert Appleby (1953–1988)

Chapter 1
Noah's New Ark:
Why should we do anything?

Every creature according to its kind

The story of Noah's Ark, in the Bible's book of Genesis, is one of the most striking and memorable in any culture. Here was a man with a mission, and it was a mission that compels our admiration and our sympathy. There may be some historical basis for the story, because there is evidence of a major flood in Mesopotamia about 6000 years ago,[1] but it is the message that is important, not the mundane facts.

Noah got the idea that he should protect the animals from danger. Where such ideas come from will be discussed shortly, but for now let us concentrate on the idea itself: the conviction, the compulsion that he should expend time and energy saving animals from destruction and looking after them until safety was assured. Not just some animals, not just the useful ones, but representatives of all animal species. It is particularly notable that he looked after animals that were thought of as 'unclean' (Box 1.1). Under Jewish law – and Noah was a Jew – certain animals such as pigs are unclean, or ceremonially impure. They cannot be eaten, and are more likely to cause revulsion than affection and protection. Practising Jews do not eat pork. Yet Noah took pigs with him on the ark: unclean animals as well as clean, wildlife as well as livestock, animals that were apparently useless as well as those that were useful.

Noah took humans as well as all the other species of animals, but he took four pairs of humans rather than one. Was he biased? Maybe so, but we should also note that those eight people had a lot of work to do for the year that they spent on the ark, feeding the animals with 'every kind of food that is to be eaten', shovelling dung and doing a thousand and one vital and

1

Box 1.1   Noah: a man with a mission

God said to Noah, 'Make yourself an ark of cypress wood. I am going to bring floodwaters on the earth to destroy all life under the heavens. But I will establish my covenant with you, and you will enter the ark. You are to bring into the ark two of all living creatures, male and female, to keep them alive with you. Two of every kind of bird, of every kind of animal and of every kind of creature that moves along the ground will come to you to be kept alive. You are to take every kind of food that is to be eaten and store it away as food for you and for them.'

Pairs of clean and unclean animals came to Noah and entered the ark, as God had commanded. Noah and his sons, Shem, Ham and Japheth, together with his wife and the wives of his three sons, entered the ark. They had with them every wild animal according to its kind, all livestock according to their kinds, every creature according to its kind and every bird according to its kind.[2]

---

unglamorous jobs of husbandry. The humans, then, were looking after all the other, non-human species of animal. Humans are animals, of course, but humans are also different from other species. In using the word 'animals' throughout this book to mean 'non-human animals' we mustn't forget either of those truths.

Is Noah's idea relevant today? Does he stand as a representative for our society's attitude to animals? Should we build a new ark? Many people obviously feel that we should: an ever-increasing number of voices can be heard saying that we should do more to protect animals and to improve their welfare. There are few dissenters – although there are those who point out difficulties and limitations in doing much about these principles, and many more who remain silent.

There are certainly parallels between Noah's story and our own. Firstly there is the element of compulsion. Just as Noah was compelled to act, so the voices of today cry that more *should* be done, not just that people who happen to feel strongly about it may do more if they wish. This compulsion will be discussed in the next sections.

A second parallel is related to the first. This compulsion, this feeling that we *should* do more, means that there will be costs involved, whether in terms of time, energy or money. We are likely to be acting against our own interests – or at least against a narrow conception of our interests in terms of short-term, direct costs and benefits. Just like Noah, we are talking about wildlife as well as livestock, animals that are less useful to us as well as those that are vital.

Thirdly, there is a sense of urgency in all this. Noah faced an event that required immediate action, and in an analogous way the issue of animal protection is gathering pace and demanding a response. Indeed, some aspects of the issue are undeniably urgent: protection of many species from extinction requires immediate attention if it is to be successful. The business of looking after species and after individual animals is therefore associated with other major problems such as environmental change, and with the perception that 'the destruction of all life under the heavens' is a real threat. Even if we leave aside protection of species and restrict our consideration to the welfare of individual animals – the main topic of this book – the urgency is still there. There are many factors that contribute, such as accelerating developments in technology and in genetic engineering, and the ready availability of information from television and the internet. This doesn't just feel like end-of-the-century despair or self-analysis, but like a real sea-change in our relationship with animals and with other aspects of the natural world.

Noah is sailing the ark of society into the twenty-first century above the flood of human population growth, technological change and environmental damage. Animals are on board, and we need to look after them (Fig. 1.1).

There are some dissenters. Some people will disagree with the emphasis of the discussion so far, or with the urgency of change. However, even those people will recognize how common are these feelings, and they will have their own limits on what they would do to animals. Almost no-one is wholly uncaring about animal welfare. Where did this consensus come from, that moral consideration of animals is appropriate? Why should anything at all be done about animal welfare?

Up the gangplank

Humans are moral beings: we consider the advantages and disadvantages of our actions to others as well as ourselves, and

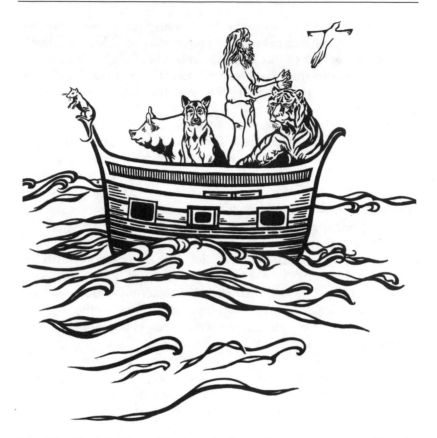

Fig. 1.1   Noah's New Ark: in today's society we must consider the welfare of all animals, on farms and in laboratories, in zoos and circuses, in our homes and in the wild.

we don't always act selfishly. Even at its simplest level this is rational and easily explained: if you think only of yourself you get less benefit from others.[3] A child hits her big brother because he's in the way. When he knocks her down she learns that this isn't the best way to get what she wants.

Furthermore, our morality doesn't just operate at that simple level: it is more than just conscious calculation of costs and benefits, and more than just subtle selfishness. Some of the child's consideration of others' feelings is subconscious, just as she may chew her food without thinking about every jaw movement. Some of this consideration is innate and some of it is learned:[4] she offers a sweet to her brother spontaneously, but learns not to hit others bigger than her (it soon doesn't even occur to her to do so). From some such behaviour she gains tangible benefits (her brother shares his sweets) and from some the benefits are more intangible (she enjoys helping her mother). However, in neither case would it be appropriate to say that the behaviour is 'really' selfish, because the benefits to her do not gainsay the effects of her behaviour for others – she really does help her mother. The emotions involved, such as enjoyment, are complex. They are associated with the bonds of affection that exist between daughter and mother, sister and brother, relatives and friends.

These aspects of human behaviour arose a long way back in our evolutionary history[5] and the 'others' concerned are not just humans. Consider the following scene (Fig. 1.2). It's a stormy day in the year 2000 BC, late in the Neolithic Stone Age. Three figures can be seen on the bank of a river in northern England: a local man, his old dog and a trader in stone axes, just arrived in the area from the flint mines in Wiltshire.[6] There is a shout, a flailing of arms and legs, then both the dog and the trader are floundering in the river. The local is safe on firm ground, a branch in his hand. Who does he save, the animal or the human?

The choice might have been more biased. The dog might have been young and still useful for hunting. The trader might have dropped his sack of valuable axes on the bank. But even without such incentives our man will surely save his dog. They have a relationship that goes back 6 or 8 years, a relationship of mutual help and attachment. The stranger is more probably an enemy than an ally. Our man doesn't analyse his dilemma, doesn't weigh up the pros and cons – and doesn't lose any sleep over the incident that night, either. He just saves his friend – who happens to be the animal, not the human.

The philosopher Mary Midgley has pointed out that when we are allocating our time, energy or money, it is understandable and reasonable that we favour those near to us – that you choose to buy your son an ice cream rather than giving the money to a charity for starving children. This doesn't mean that you should give all your resources to your son and none to charity, but nor should you be expected to be completely impartial. And 'near to us' is not a concept with neat concentric circles – family at the middle, friends in the next circle, other humans further out and animals beyond all humans (Fig. 1.3). Animals are often part of the family in this sense, and it is understandable and reasonable that we should give some of our time, energy and money, some

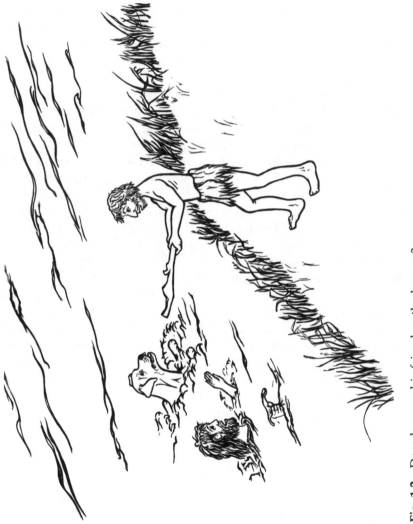

Fig. 1.2 Does he save his friend or the human?

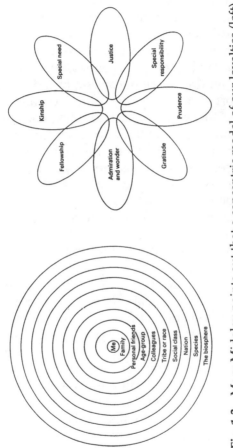

Fig. 1.3 Mary Midgley points out that a concentric model of our loyalties (left) does not work: some groupings are more important for some purposes, some for others. Instead we must consider various kinds of claims (right), and these may concern animals as well as humans.[7]

of our help and some of our affection to animals rather than humans.[7]

As society developed after the last ice age and humans domesticated sheep and goats, cattle and pigs, this concern for animals must have been important. No doubt the predominant factor in the relationship was human benefit, but there must always have been care for the animals and limits to mistreatment.[8] Then as now, the shepherd who cared for his sheep found them easier to handle, and kept more of them alive, than another who literally couldn't care less.

Caring for animals was associated with another important tendency: an understanding of animal behaviour. Understanding the behaviour of a wolf who might eat you or a deer you might eat had been important for millennia. Now you also needed to know where your cattle would graze and when your pigs would mate. Domestic animals are not a random selection from all the wild animals available. They are those that were both useful and easy to domesticate. One of the factors that affected both the usefulness and the ease of domestication was whether we could understand their behaviour – whether we could communicate. Juliet Clutton-Brock is an archaeologist who has taken a particular interest in domestication. She points out that dogs are descended from wolves, not African hunting dogs:

> The hunting dog ... is a most highly social carnivore that lives and hunts in packs but ... social behaviour is more dependent on the mutual regurgitation of food and less on communication by facial expression and posture than in the wolf. So that if man is not prepared to receive the regurgitated offerings of a hunting dog into his own mouth his powers of communication with the animal are going to be limited. Whereas there can be such a close empathy between man and dog that if a puppy is reared amongst a human family that smiles a lot the dog will actually mimic this expression of pleasure by a sideways grin of the lips and muscles around the mouth.[6]

The idea that dogs imitate smiling from humans is probably wrong, but the general point that we communicate more readily with domestic dogs than with hunting dogs is well made. The understanding of animals is one of the elements of animal welfare that will be covered in the next two chapters.

Today there is cultural variation in concern for animals.

Concern is strongest and most widespread in northern and western Europe, and in areas such as North America and Australasia, presumably because emigration from Europe to those areas led to cultural similarities. Ironically, this increased concern apparently developed among people who were less involved with animals than in other areas. The UK and The Netherlands, for example, were more industrialized than many other countries, and pressure for animal protection largely came from city dwellers rather than from those actually involved in farming.[9]

Other cultural differences are more difficult to explain. In oriental countries such as Japan there is less concern for animal welfare than in the West, but more about the killing of animals. So while many families have their own rice paddies, few rear animals such as ducks that they would have to kill themselves. Sick animals are sometimes allowed to die slowly rather than being put out of their misery, because people are reluctant actually to kill them. Some of this is religious, part of the attitudes to life and death of Buddhism and Shintoism, but it is still relevant to ask where these attitudes came from. Perhaps the ecology of early humans in areas where Buddhism developed was different to that in Europe. Both the influence of wild animals such as wolves and dependence on domestic animals may have been very different indeed. However, some cultural variation may be essentially due to chance, may be 'purely' cultural. People's ideas are influenced by many factors (including the pronouncements of particular individuals such as Buddha), and so societies may grow apart by 'cultural drift' as well as in ways that are functional.

So much for history and speculation on history. Are attitudes to animals rational or consistent today?

Wanted on voyage

What use is philosophy? The question is often asked, but philosophers have done more to promote discussion of animal welfare and animal protection than anyone else, whether scientists, politicians or activists. Peter Singer, author of *Animal Liberation*,[10] and Tom Regan, who wrote *The Case For Animal Rights*,[11] produced clear, reasoned arguments. They also produced massive publicity, partly because the titles of their books were readily turned into slogans. However, they also caused some confusion, because they took different approaches to the subject and came up with different conclusions. We shall see below that most people actually follow a mixed approach, with elements of the first two (Table 1.1). This hybrid approach can be fairly coherent but does lead to some tensions.

One major approach in moral philosophy, or ethics, concentrates mostly or wholly on the *consequences* of our actions.[12] Whether you tripped over the cat or deliberately kicked him is not the primary fact. What matters most is that the cat was hurt. The best-known form of this approach is utilitarianism: the idea that we should act so as to produce the greatest good (or utility) for the greatest number of individuals. Singer is a utilitarian. His particular contribution was to stress that when we reckon up the good and bad consequences of our actions, consequences for animals must be given equal weight to those for humans unless there are impartial grounds for doing otherwise. If you claim that you kicked the cat to relieve your feelings that is a poor excuse: you are valuing a small benefit to yourself more than the large cost to the cat. Singer argued persuasively that humans have unthinkingly valued benefits to humans more than costs to animals (he called this *speciesism* by analogy with racism and sexism) and that this led to vivisection and factory farming. His form of utilitarianism is a powerful argument against mistreatment. It is not, however, an argument against killing. Singer believes, for example, that if a pig has a good life and is killed humanely, death is not a significant harm done to the pig because the pig is not aware of what it is losing. Awareness will be considered further in Chapter 3.

Few people are pure utilitarians. Most feel that the pleasure of 20 000 people in an amphitheatre did not justify the suffering of a gladiator in Roman times, and many feel that it does not justify the suffering of a bull today either.

A second ethical approach, then, is that there are some things we should do, and some things we should not do, regardless of good or bad consequences. Torturing monkeys is wrong, even if it is part of a programme to produce a new medicine. This approach leads to the dual concepts of duties and rights. Regan suggested that these include human duties to animals or animal rights. According to this argument, animals have the right not to be harmed, which includes not being killed. Regan believes that a pig is indeed harmed by being killed, and that we should therefore not kill animals for food.

Table 1.1 Animal ethics

Approach	Emphasis on consequences of actions	Emphasis on actions being right or wrong in themselves	Mixed approach
Terms used	Consequentialism Utilitarianism Extrinsic issues	Duties Rights Intrinsic issues	
Examples	Singer extends utilitarianism to include consequences for animals: 'speciesism' is wrong	Religions argue for human duties Regan argues for animal rights	Sandøe suggests many people have hybrid views
Common conclusions	Animal welfare should be improved. Humane killing may be acceptable	Animal welfare should be improved. Killing is rarely acceptable	DeGrazia: Don't cause significant suffering for the sake of enjoyment.[17] Strength of conclusions on welfare and killing varies between people and between animal species

Many other aspects of ethics come under this second, broad heading, including religious views. Noah felt he had a duty to animals, and believed very clearly that his duty was given to him by God. Many religious people today have the same view, that we have a duty to care for God's kingdom, including his animals. Many other people take a similar position in relation to nature or to the environment, either because of similar arguments about duties and rights or because of other ethical frameworks. They feel that we ought to care for the environment, including animals. This ecological perspective has also produced an additional focus for ethics: it suggests that we may have duties to protect animal species, as well as the individual members of those species.

There is room for debate in all this. Perhaps most important, the theory of rights leaves us with many difficult decisions. Does the mouse in my kitchen have the right not to be killed? If I have the right to kill that mouse, why not another in a medical experiment? Furthermore, some philosophers feel that the idea of animal rights is actually of no practical value, partly because animals can't speak for themselves,[13] and that we should concentrate on human duties. This doesn't mean that they are against animal protection. On the contrary, they argue that human duties include improvement of animal welfare. Even Michael Leahy, who wrote a diatribe called *Against Liberation*, criticizes the conditions on intensive farms and in barren zoo enclosures.[14]

There is also another element of confusion. The term 'animal rights' is sometimes used in a loose sense to refer to the whole issue of animal protection, rather than in the formal sense proposed by Regan. Peter Singer himself is sometimes associated with 'animal rights' in this loose sense, in phrases like 'father of the animal rights movement', adding to the confusion. Singer supports animal protection but not animal rights.

Setting this aside, what do the two approaches have in common? Simply, both argue that we should do more for animal welfare, although they disagree on how we should do the reckoning up. Other conclusions differ. One major disagreement is on whether killing animals for human benefit is generally permissible. Singer says that it is, if benefits outweigh costs. Regan's emphasis on rights suggests that it isn't.

However, most people do not follow Singer or Regan in attempting complete consistency in their ethical approach. Our minds don't work like that. The ways in which we think have developed through evolution, history and our own lifetimes as outlined in the previous section. We react to situations and problems as they arise without being completely consistent. Indeed, it is impossible to be completely consistent.[15] Mary Midgley says, 'The idea that morality could be reduced to a single basic form is a foolish one'.[16] So what do we do? We adopt a more-or-less coherent set of ideas that arise partly from our historical and social background and partly from reasoned argument.[17] The Danish philosopher Peter Sandøe suggests that:

> A hybrid view which is attractive to many people combines elements from utilitarianism and the animal rights view. One version of this would say that there are certain things that one may not do to animals, no matter how beneficial the consequences, for example causing the animals to experience intense suffering. As long as we abstain from these things we can, on this view, reason as a utilitarian would do. For example, killing of animals or causing them mild distress or inconvenience may be allowed if sufficiently good consequences follow.[18]

Other people come to a different balance of views. For example, the American Bernard Rollin suggests that society is moving towards acceptance of ideas associated with animal rights.[19] People don't necessarily believe in animal rights as such, but an increasing number dislike the idea of killing animals.

So most of us tend to tackle questions on an individual basis while avoiding inconsistency to a greater or lesser extent but not completely. This approach does not avoid problems and tensions (discussed in Chapter 4), but recognition that it is a reasonable stance has at least two major advantages. Firstly it reflects how people actually think, rather than painting them into a corner. If you read *Animal Liberation* and *The Case For Animal Rights* and agreed with most of both, you're not alone. Secondly, it offers the possibility of avoiding rigid positions. It allows discussion between people who disagree. It rejects the 'football match' between utilitarians and animal rightists.[16] It allows consensus.

A very widespread consensus, among philosophers and many other people, is that we should do more for animal welfare. As Mahatma Gandhi said:

> The greatness of a nation and its moral progress can be judged by the way its animals are treated.

Who is at the helm?

It is easy to point the finger of blame. Farmers are greedy, scientists are heartless and politicians are short-sighted. Are they really? As the bumper sticker puts it, 'Don't criticize farmers with your mouth full.'

There are certainly some farmers, some scientists, some politicians who fit these stereotypes; they deserve their share of the blame and they get it, both in society and in the later chapters of this book. However, the broad picture is not so simple. Most farmers would like to improve conditions for their animals, but they would go out of business if they did. Profit margins are small in farming and if farmers increased their costs they could not compete in the open market. Most farmers are not rich: they live on an overdraft, on a knife-edge between prosperity and bankruptcy. Imagine a farmer going to the bank and asking for a loan to increase the size of his cow shed. 'How much more income from your cows do you expect?' asks the banker. 'None' answers the farmer. 'Goodbye' says the banker.

If all farmers could agree to improve conditions, conditions could be improved. But the free market doesn't work like that. They could never get 100% agreement, and anyway agreements like that are criticized as price-fixing monopolies. The situation is also made more complex by international trade. Even if all the dairy farmers in The Netherlands agreed to give their cows more space they would still lose business, because of cheap milk coming into the country from outside.

So this is a matter for legislation. The public say to the farmers, 'Be nice to your cows' and they say to the politicians, 'Tell the farmers what to do.' The farmers say to the politicians, 'Give us a level playing field for our cows!' The politicians say to the public, 'Surely you don't want to pay more for your milk?'

Who is responsible for improving animal welfare? The answer, clearly, is all of us. There is a communal responsibility, as indicated by Gandhi's comment about nations, and all the members of the community have an individual responsibility too.

In saying that we should do more about animal welfare, 'we' includes people with special responsibility, such as farmers, scientists and politicians. It includes those with special interest, such as certain philosophers, welfarists and scientists who study welfare, and it includes the general public.

This is not the place to discuss all possible duties on animal welfare, for each of these groups. Many such duties will come up in later chapters, but one area may serve as an example, the area of communication.

Farmers who keep animals and scientists who do experiments on animals are still, in general, too defensive about criticism. If there are good reasons for what they do, they should say so, and co-operate with those who want to see improvements. There is much more room for statements like 'Yes, I would like to wean piglets at 5 weeks old rather than 4; can you help me to make that economically viable?', 'Yes, I would like to experiment on cell cultures instead of mice but it will cost more in the short term; how can I raise the money?' Farms, laboratories and other institutions with nothing to be ashamed of should hold more open days.[20] Those responsible for animals could do more to take the initiative rather than just responding to demands. Politicians need to listen. Sir Colin Spedding, chairman of the UK's Farm Animal Welfare Council, points out that 'It is very important to listen to moderate views and not, as so often happens, brush them aside. Ignoring moderates can generate extremists.'[21]

Many of those who are activists in one sense or other see their main responsibility as obtaining and providing information. This book is a part of that process. However, people with particular concern for welfare could still do more to communicate. Welfare organizations could talk to farmers' unions, to zoo directors, to hunters. Philosophers writing on animal protection could find out more about what actually happens on farms, rather than just decrying the principles of factory farming and vivisection. Welfare scientists could write more newspaper articles, rather than just papers in obscure journals.

Members of the general public vary in their perceptions. Indeed, all the above specialists are also members of the public. Everyone has responsibilities concerning animals, as discussed above, so they should be receptive to information on animal welfare and should not ignore that information when they have it. There is a model traditionally called the Three Wise Monkeys, representing the principles: see no evil, hear no evil, speak no evil. They should instead be called the Three Irresponsible Monkeys (Fig. 1.4). Avoiding knowledge about things that are wrong, and staying silent about them once they are known, are actions that help to perpetuate wrongdoing. Informing ourselves and then speaking out are actions that help to combat evil. If you do not know how veal calves are raised, it may be reasonable to

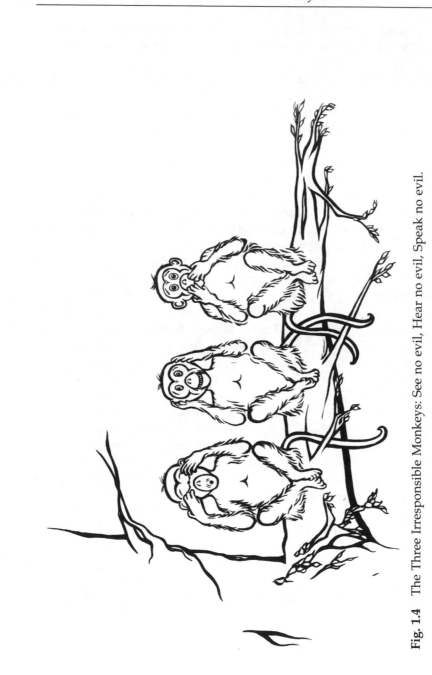

Fig. 1.4   The Three Irresponsible Monkeys: See no evil, Hear no evil, Speak no evil.

eat veal. Once you have been told, you ought to take that into account. There may also be a duty to obtain more information. Read the rest of this book.

It is important that we let our views be known: a consensus cannot otherwise be obtained. As Michael Reiss (who is both a scientist and a priest) points out, a consensus is not just majority voting, 'It should be based on reason, should take into account long established practices of ethical reasoning and be open to refutation and the possibility of change.'[22] In other words, these issues must be discussed fully, publicly and repeatedly.

Conclusions

- Concern for animals arose a long way back in our evolutionary history and is a rational and reasonable response to the animals who share our world.
- While there is cultural variation across the world, in many countries there is increasing concern for animal welfare, on farms and in laboratories, in zoos and circuses, in our homes and in the wild.
- Moral philosophers offer frameworks for the ethics of animal protection, such as utilitarianism and animal rights. Most people follow a mixed approach, tackling questions on an individual basis and avoiding inconsistency to a greater or lesser extent.
- We are all responsible for animal welfare: those closely involved (such as farmers, scientists and politicians), those with special interest (certain philosophers, welfarists and scientists who study welfare) and the general public.
- Communication on matters concerning animal welfare is vital. Informing ourselves, and letting our views be known, are central to achieving both consensus and change.

References

1. Keller, W. (1956) *The Bible as History*. Hodder & Stoughton, London.
2. Genesis, Chapters 6–7, *New International Translation of the Bible*. Hodder & Stoughton, London. (The quotation is abridged.)
3. Parfit, D. (1984) *Reasons and Persons*. Oxford University Press, Oxford.
4. Barkow, J.H., Cosmides, L. & Tooby, J. (eds) (1992) *The Adapted Mind: Evolutionary Psychology and the Generation of Culture*. Oxford University Press, Oxford.

5. Ridley, M. (1996) *The Origins of Virtue*. Viking, London; de Waal, F. (1996) *Good Natured: The Origins of Right and Wrong in Humans and Other Animals*. Harvard University Press, Cambridge, Mass., USA.
6. Clutton-Brock, J. (1987) *A Natural History of Domesticated Mammals*. British Museum (Natural History), London.
7. Midgley, M. (1983) *Animals and Why They Matter*. University of Georgia Press, Athens, Ga., USA.
8. Budiansky, S. (1992) *The Covenant of the Wild: Why Animals Chose Domestication*. Weidenfeld & Nicolson, London.
9. Appleby, M.C., Hughes, B.O. & Elson, H.A. (1992) *Poultry Production Systems: Behaviour, Management and Welfare*. CAB International, Wallingford, UK.
10. Singer, P. (1975) *Animal Liberation*. New York Review of Books, New York.
11. Regan, T. (1983) *The Case for Animal Rights*. University of California Press, Berkeley.
12. Anon. (1980) Consequentialism. In *The Oxford Dictionary of Philosophy* (ed. S. Blackburn). Oxford University Press, Oxford.
13. Carruthers, P. (1992) *The Animals Issue: Moral Theory in Practice*. Cambridge University Press, Cambridge.
14. Leahy, M.P.T. (1991) *Against Liberation: Putting Animals in Perspective*. Routledge, London.
15. Williams, B. (1972) *Morality: An Introduction to Ethics*. Cambridge University Press, Cambridge.
16. Midgley, M. (1986) Letter to the Editors. *Between the Species*, **2**, 195–6.
17. DeGrazia, D. (1996) *Taking Animals Seriously: Mental Life and Moral Status*. Cambridge University Press, Cambridge.
18. Sandøe, P., Crisp R. & Holtug, N. (1997) Ethics. In *Animal Welfare* (eds M.C. Appleby & B.O. Hughes), pp. 3–17. CAB International, Wallingford, UK.
19. Rollin, B.E. (1995) *The Frankenstein Syndrome: Ethical and Social Issues in the Genetic Engineering of Animals*. Cambridge University Press, Cambridge.
20. Clifton, M. (1996) Primate behavior and the research controversy. Talk presented to Cornell University Students for the Ethical Treatment of Animals.
21. Spedding, C. (1996) Overview of animal welfare in farming. In *Welfare Problems of Food Animals and Horses. 2. The Economics of Food Animal Welfare* (eds A. Suckling, A.J. Higgins & J.F. Wade). Animal Health Trust, British Veterinary Association Animal Welfare Foundation and Royal Society for Prevention of Cruelty to Animals, UK.
22. Reiss, M. (1997) Ethical issues. In *Genetic Engineering in Food Production* (ed. Lord Soulsby), pp. 165–175. Royal Society of Medicine Press, London.

Chapter 2
Humans, animals and machines: Understanding animal welfare

It all seems obvious

There are dozens of meetings every year about animal welfare, among scientists, philosophers, theologians, politicians and interested members of the public. There are discussions, conferences and books about the subject. All of these spend an extraordinary amount of time discussing the question, what is animal welfare? This strikes many other people as a complete waste of time. The question has probably never occurred to them, and when they hear it the answer seems obvious. Chapter 1 talked about animal welfare without defining it: about caring for animals, preventing suffering, improving their living conditions. This all seems self-evident, so the talking-shops are clearly useless. Can't the experts just get on with improving animal welfare?

The answer – this is the scientist's answer to almost every question – is, yes and no. We can make progress without definitions. We can clamp down on cruelty and deal with the worst abuses. We can study animals and their responses to the environment, find out about the causes of disease and injury, devise ways of preventing them. David Fraser, Professor of Animal Welfare at the University of Vancouver, says that welfare scientists give too much attention to the big picture and not enough to the details. They can't see the trees for the wood:

> Instead of trying to 'measure' animal welfare, scientists should see their task as identifying, solving and preventing animal welfare problems.[1]

On the other hand, suppose we say to farmers, 'Improve the welfare of your animals.' The farmers ask, 'What do you

19

mean by welfare?' To some extent this is defensive manoeuvring: they don't want to change their ways so they throw up legalistic obstacles of definition. But to some extent it is a reasonable question. A major reason for this is that different aspects of welfare are contradictory. For example, more and more UK pig farmers have moved their pigs outdoors over the last few years. The mother sows have more freedom but they sometimes get cold, and more of the piglets become ill and die. If the most important aspect of welfare is freedom, more farmers should move their pigs outside. If warmth and health of the piglets are more important, perhaps outdoor farmers should move their animals back in. Such contradictions will be considered in more detail in later chapters, but for now here is another example. David Fraser and colleagues tell the following story (Fig. 2.1):

> Two dog owners met one day to walk their dogs together. One owner had grown up in a small family that valued health, safety and orderly, disciplined behaviour. The dog of this owner received regular veterinary care, two meals a day of low-fat dog food, and was walked on a leash. The other owner had grown up in a large community that valued conviviality, sharing of resources and close contact with the natural world. This dog (the owner's third – the first two had been killed by cars) had burrs in its coat, was fed generously but sporadically, and had never worn a collar in its life. Each owner, judging quality of life from very different viewpoints, felt sorry for the other's dog.[2]

So pig farmers and dog owners may well ask, What do you mean by welfare?

There is another, related reason for the question. Where definite decisions are required (move pigs outdoors, ban the battery cage, stop vivisection), they need a very firm foundation or there will be endless argument. This is particularly clear with legislation. For a law to be acceptable to the people to whom it applies, credible to the inspectors policing it and reasonable to the magistrates dealing with cases in the courts, it needs a clear basis. So the aim of this chapter is to provide a well-founded basis for the understanding of animal welfare.

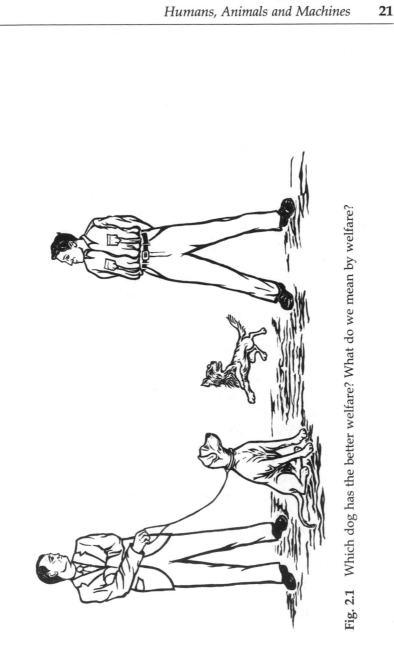

Fig. 2.1 Which dog has the better welfare? What do we mean by welfare?

Animal machines

First, though, a step backwards is necessary. There is a theoretical argument that there is actually no such thing as animal welfare. The seventeenth century philosopher René Descartes is credited with the idea that animals are machines, like clocks, which do not feel anything at all.[3] This idea must be explained before it is set aside, because it is not as ridiculous as it appears and needs to be answered.

We can train a worm to turn left. If we place it repeatedly in a Y-shaped tube with food in the left arm of the Y and salt (which is bad for it) in the right arm, after a while it will turn left more often than right. The nerve signals that control the muscles change over time, so that they cause the head to swing left at the junction. The physiology can account for the behaviour without any complications such as the worm feeling pleasure when it eats or pain when it gets salt on its skin. So, the argument says, the dog who wags her tail or cowers with her tail between her legs is behaving in the same, mechanical way, without any emotions or feelings involved.

This argument need not detain us. There is no known way that it can be disproved: we cannot prove definitively that animals feel pleasure or pain. However, we cannot prove that other humans feel pleasure or pain either. I do not know for certain that my next-door neighbour has feelings. He acts as I do in circumstances similar to those that I would like or dislike, showing expressions, making sounds and using words that suggest pleasure or pain, but he might still be play-acting, or showing behaviour automatically without any underlying feelings. I cannot know whether he feels the same as I do. Nobody except him can know for sure that he feels anything at all. Despite this, I am not allowed to punch him on the nose. We decide as a society that people should not be allowed to do certain things to each other, and there is a consensus in society – as discussed in Chapter 1 – that people should not be allowed to do certain things to animals either. The question is, what things? This consensus assumes that animal welfare does exist.

In the seventeenth century, some people agreed with Descartes and carried out extensive vivisection on fully conscious animals.[4] Some tendency to a similar belief may have lingered on and contributed to the establishment of factory farming – to the treatment of animals *as if* they were machines. This was implied by the title of Ruth Harrison's influential book on that subject, borrowed as a heading for this section, *Animal Machines*,[5] but I know of only two scientists who have supported this argument in recent years. Bob Bermond is a psychologist, whose ideas will be outlined in the next chapter.[6] John Kennedy was a zoologist (he died in 1996), who argued that we cannot know whether animals have feelings. He then made the jump to believing that they do not have feelings – perhaps influenced by the fact that he worked all his life on insects. Such people are in a very small minority, and if they want to convert the world to their way of thinking the burden of proof is on them. Furthermore, their views have limited implications in practice. Kennedy said of scientists that:

> If they assume that animals do not feel pain, or have doubts about it, they can nevertheless quite sincerely support legal measures and professional codes of conduct to prevent animals being treated in ways that most people believe are unkind, because such treatments arouse feelings of pity and revulsion in most scientists too.[7]

As we said, this is a theoretical argument. Animal welfare exists in practice, even if (and it is a big *if*) not in theory.

Kennedy does, though, make an important point. Many people assume, more or less frequently and more or less unconsciously, that animals think and feel as humans do. This assumption is called anthropomorphism,[8] and it can be conveyed by the idea that animals, far from being machines, are little humans.

Little humans

It is not uncommon for someone living on his own with a dog to express the idea that 'She understands every word I say'. He may not mean it literally, and he doesn't treat the dog as if she was a human, but there is a danger that thinking of her as if she is almost a human means that he will not treat her appropriately for a dog either.

Anthropomorphism can lead to problems. Jeffrey Masson visited an Indian game reserve:

> After a mile or so we came across a herd of about ten elephants, including small calves, peacefully grazing ... I walked closer, halting about twenty feet away. One large elephant looked

toward me and flapped his ears. Knowing nothing about elephants, I had no idea this was a warning. Blissfully ignorant, as if I were in a zoo or in the presence of Babar or some other story-book elephant, I felt it was time to commune with the elephants ... I called out *'Bhoh, gajendra'* – Greetings, Lord of the Elephants.

The elephant trumpeted; for a second I thought it was his return greeting. Then his sudden, surprisingly agile turn and thunderous charge in my direction made it all too clear that he did not participate in my elephant fantasies. I was aghast to see a two-ton animal come hurtling toward me ... I turned and ran wildly.[9]

Most mistakes are not so dramatic. Yet some people try to keep cats on a vegetarian diet, mindless of the fact that food suitable for humans may be unsuitable for carnivores with different dietary requirements.

Mistakes also occur when people take an anthropomorphic view of the welfare of captive animals. It used to be common in zoos and menageries to keep lions in small cages, where they would lie motionless for most of the time, waiting for the next meal. People used to say, 'What a shame. They're yearning to roam free.' So when Whipsnade Zoo, north of London, had space and money they built a large paddock for their lions. The lions continued to lie motionless for most of the time, waiting for the next meal. With the hindsight of numerous television documentaries, we now know that this is what they do in the wild too. This is not to say that welfare was satisfactory in the earlier small cages, but it does suggest that inactivity – which would be boring for humans – is insufficient evidence for welfare problems in lions.

So the criticism of a battery cage that simply says, 'I wouldn't like being in a cage like that, so we shouldn't do it to hens' is ill-founded. Hens are not little humans.

This does not mean, of course, that we should swing back to the other extreme and treat hens as machines. We can certainly make some conclusions about their welfare. Furthermore, some of those conclusions may be based on *careful* anthropomorphism.

Mary Midgley points out that anthropomorphism has been demonized in science.[8] People like Kennedy have emphasized that animals do not think exactly as humans do. This is undeniable. However, they have then claimed that we cannot draw any conclusions at all about animal behaviour from our own experience.[10] This is untenable. In Chapter 1 there was a mention of Stone Age people and their understanding of the behaviour of a wolf who might eat them. Obviously they used their own view of the world to predict what the wolf might do. Obviously the prediction wasn't perfect, and they quickly learned how to improve it; equally obviously they did better than if they had started with no assumptions at all about the wolf's behaviour. Anthropomorphism is something of a dirty word among scientists, but Midgley suggests that what might be called partial anthropomorphism is both unavoidable and invaluable. So we should go along with Kennedy in avoiding uncritical anthropomorphism, but also avoid the blindfold that he put on to prevent it.

We can and must walk a middle path between uncritical anthropomorphism and viewing animals as machines. We can and must reach a realistic understanding of animal welfare.

Back to basics

Some of the meetings and discussions mentioned above have produced definitions of welfare. Unfortunately, most of these don't add much to understanding. For example, in 1965 a committee led by Professor Rogers Brambell reported to the UK Government on the welfare of farm animals. It said that welfare is 'A wide term that embraces both the physical and mental well-being of the animal.'[11] So welfare is well-being: that doesn't help much. In fact, the terms welfare and well-being are generally (and certainly in this book) regarded as synonyms.

Other definitions have more-or-less been lists of concepts thought to be relevant to welfare. For example, in talking about outdoor pigs earlier in the chapter, three aspects of welfare came up: freedom, warmth and health. Here are some other concepts that regularly arise in discussion, in no particular order: comfort, happiness, lack of suffering, care and attention, natural environment.

Some of the items in a list like this may be contradictory, as we have already noted. Thus many people believe that animals should receive care and attention to ensure their health, but be kept in conditions as natural as possible. Furthermore, such lists tend to include both factors that affect welfare (like care and attention) and the responses of the animals to such factors (like happiness). So how can we move on from such an unstructured 'shopping-list' approach?

The rest of this chapter provides a logical framework for ideas about animal welfare by outlining three categories for animal responses that people think are important. This framework has been suggested by two professors of animal welfare in Canada, David Fraser and Ian Duncan, and their work[12] forms the basis for what follows. The first category concerns animal feelings, such as happiness and lack of suffering. The second involves bodily matters such as health. The third concerns the question of whether animals lead natural lives. They can be summarized by the phrase: mind, body and nature. This is very similar to the idea of mind, body and spirit in humans, especially as the concept of spirit is close to that of human nature.

There are two other points to make before moving on, which are matters of general agreement among those working on animal welfare. First, 'Welfare is a characteristic of an animal, not something given to it'.[13] This runs counter to a perception held by some people that animal welfare refers only to our effects on animals.

Secondly, welfare is not all-or-nothing. Originally 'welfare' meant 'well-being, happiness' – literally 'a state of faring well'[14] – but it is now used to mean a state that can vary from good to bad. It makes sense to talk of 'poor welfare' or of 'improving welfare', concepts that are vital and for which there is no other word, just as it makes sense to talk of 'bad luck' or of 'poor health'.

Having considered the background, we shall now go on to consider animal feelings.

Through animal eyes

Implicit in most of the discussion so far – for example, in the discussion of anthropomorphism – is the idea that welfare concerns the perceptions or feelings of animals. You wonder whether your canary is happy. Is he bored and lonely in his cage? Would he be happier in the wild, or would he be hungry, cold and frightened?

The idea that feelings are central to welfare was implicit in the writing of Jeremy Bentham in the eighteenth century and has been re-affirmed recently by Marian Dawkins in the UK and Ian Duncan in Canada (Box 2.1).

Box 2.1   Welfare and animal minds

Jeremy Bentham	The question is not, Can they *reason*? nor, Can they *talk*? but, Can they *suffer*?[15]
Marian Dawkins	To be concerned about animal welfare is to be concerned with the subjective feelings of animals, particularly the unpleasant subjective feelings of suffering and pain.[16]
Ian Duncan	It is generally agreed that welfare is a term which cannot be applied sensibly to the lower animals or to plants but only to sentient animals. Since 'sentient' means capable of feelings, the argument is developed that welfare is solely dependent on what animals feel.[17]

What can we learn about animal feelings? To what extent can we see through animal eyes? To repeat what was said above, there is no known way that we can *prove anything* about animal feelings. However, we have plenty of evidence.[18] We can use this just as the jury in a court of law uses evidence to come to a conclusion, when there is no cast-iron proof of guilt or innocence. There are two sorts of evidence: evidence about whether animals are happy, and evidence about what they want.[19]

Some evidence about whether animals are happy comes from their behaviour. In some cases this evidence is positive, but positive evidence tends to be patchy and difficult to interpret. Young animals that are playing look happy, and so do most pet dogs when the people who live with them arrive home. Surprisingly, there are few examples of adult animals looking unequivocally happy – yet to suggest that they are rarely happy would seem too strong a conclusion. Dogs and cats are a special case, because they have been selected and trained to go on showing juvenile behaviour.[20] However, while it is common to talk about contented cows, grazing in the sunshine, this is more likely to reflect a human observer's view that 'This is how things ought to be, and all's right with the world' than a genuine judgement that the cows are happy, doing what they're doing. In other words, this is an area where uncritical anthropomorphism is rife. Sometimes mistakes are fairly clear. A visitor to the zoo sees chimpanzees tumbling over one another and one baring its teeth in what looks like a smile. Perhaps they are playing. No, closer inspection shows that this is a young male, being beaten up by an elder. Its expression is known to behavioural scientists as a fear-grin.[21] There are other examples where we can conclude very little about the feelings associated with behaviour. Does the fact that your canary sings in its cage mean that it is happy? We have no idea.

More of the behavioural evidence about animal feelings is negative. There are many types of behaviour that suggest animals are suffering. For example, young male farm animals are often castrated without anaesthetic. Piglets scream during the operation,[22] and lambs stamp their feet and stand and lie awkwardly afterwards.[23] It seems reasonable to conclude that the animals are in pain.[24] This evidence is also useful for comparisons. One method of castration causes less such behaviour than another, so it may be concluded that it is less painful.[23]

Information about problems also comes from *abnormal behaviour* – behaviour that is rare or absent except in particular circumstances. The clearest example is the stereotyped actions shown by some zoo animals, such as polar bears pacing in circles (Fig. 2.2), and some farm animals, such as sows biting or mouthing the bars of their pen. Research on this behaviour, including physiological measurements from the animals, suggests that in most cases the animals have been through a period of stress that caused the behaviour to become established, or are stressed now, or both.[25]

Physiological measurements are also useful on their own, particularly for comparisons. Ian Duncan and colleagues measured the heart rate of broiler chickens that were being caught by hand or by machine. Heart rate went up in both groups, and they assumed that the birds were frightened. It returned to normal more quickly in the latter group, so they concluded that it was actually less frightening for a chicken to be picked up by a machine than by a person.[26] Incidentally the word 'chicken' is used here and throughout the book to mean a domestic fowl of any age, as distinct from the word 'chick' which means a young one. There is no other convenient word which can mean either a hen or a cockerel.

Behaviour also provides evidence on what animals want, and hence again on their feelings.[27] The cats seen on television advertisements, choosing the appropriate catfood and turning

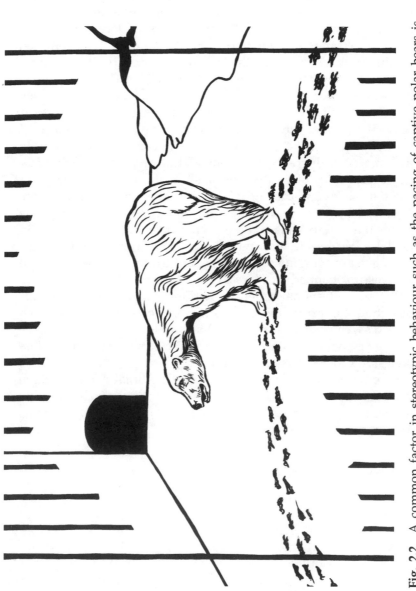

Fig. 2.2 A common factor in stereotypic behaviour such as the pacing of captive polar bears is prevention of foraging behaviour, and it may be associated with stress or frustration.

their noses up at inferior brands, are giving us just such evidence (or at least, they are doing so if we can trust the advertisements). This sort of choice is called a *preference test*, and such tests have been used in practical ways like improving the design of loading ramps for animal trucks.[28] What is more, we can assess the strength of animal preferences. For example, it is common farming practice to restrict the food of sows to stop them getting too fat. Do they get used to this restriction? No. There are many lines of evidence to suggest strongly that they are hungry. They show hyperactivity at feeding time, and they eat more than their ration if they get the chance. With colleagues at Edinburgh, I trained pigs that were fed on standard commercial rations to push a panel, operating a machine that delivered small addi-tional quantities of food. They pushed the panel hundreds of times in a 20 minute test.[29] The conclusion that they were chronically hungry was widely accepted, and was one of the factors that led to stalls and tethers for sows being phased out in the UK, because it was agreed that preventing such hungry animals from foraging was unacceptable. Stalls and tethers will soon also be banned in the rest of the EU (Fig. 2.3).

Preference tests have their limitations – for example, animals may choose options which give them a short-term benefit (such as food sweetened with saccharin) but no long-term advantage – but they provide evidence about animal feelings that can be taken alongside other forms of evidence.

So to some extent we can see through animal eyes. We have made some progress in interpreting their feelings and identifying problems – although less in being able to conclude that problems are absent and that they are happy.

If it works, don't fix it

Most people agree that welfare concerns animal feelings. Many people, though, think that progress in understanding and judg-ing feelings is not enough. It will be a long time, if ever, before we know how an animal feels about being healthy or ill. Mean-while, these people say, we must study health itself, and other aspects of how well the animal's body works or functions. Other approaches to this issue are possible, too. Barry Hughes and Peter Curtis, vets working on welfare, say 'Many veterinarians think that taking care of an animal's physical health will auto-matically take care of its mental health.'[31] Furthermore, an

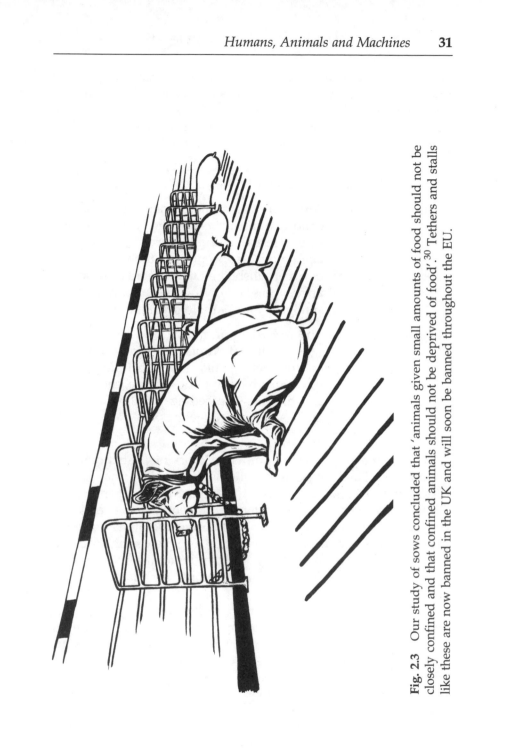

Fig. 2.3 Our study of sows concluded that 'animals given small amounts of food should not be closely confined and that confined animals should not be deprived of food'.[30] Tethers and stalls like these are now banned in the UK and will soon be banned throughout the EU.

animal may have an illness of which it is unaware – which doesn't yet cause it to suffer – and some people think that this nevertheless reduces its welfare.[32] These ideas have been expressed by two other scientists working on welfare, Harold Gonyou in Canada and Donald Broom in the UK (Box 2.2).

Box 2.2   Welfare and animal bodies

Harold Gonyou	Although the animal's perception of its condition must serve as the basis for well-being, research in this area is only just beginning. At the present time much can be accomplished by using more traditional approaches involving behavioural, physiological and pathological studies.[33]
Donald Broom	The welfare of an individual is its state as regards its attempts to cope with its environment. This state includes how much it is having to do to cope, the extent to which it is succeeding or failing to cope, and its associated feelings.[34]

How do we judge that an animal is 'working', functioning or coping well? Firstly, we can ask whether it is healthy. Injuries and diseases are commonly regarded as among the most important welfare problems. They can often be prevented. For example, a considerable amount is known about design and management to prevent injury and disease in farm animals, where such problems reduce profit.[35] However, it has to be said that this knowledge is not always put into practice: the economic benefit may not be sufficient.

If animals are well, they are not just healthy. They are eating and drinking regularly. Young animals are growing well. Adults, given the opportunity, are reproducing successfully. Cows are producing milk and hens are producing eggs when appropriate.

As with feelings, not all these factors are useful as positive evidence that all is well. Egg production provides a good example. We have selected hens over many generations for the number of eggs they lay, and a hen has egg production as a priority that overrides many other aspects of her biology. She goes on producing eggs, which need a lot of calcium for the shells, even if her bones are weak from loss of calcium.[36] So the fact that she is laying well does not prove that her welfare is good. On the other hand, these factors may be useful as *negative* evidence, evidence of poor welfare. If a hen lays fewer eggs than usual or stops laying altogether, there is probably something wrong.

Apart from the tangible signs of things going wrong, one other major concept is commonly used in this context: stress. Stress is sometimes deduced from behaviour or from physical effects such as failure to grow, but more often from physiological measurements. Certain physiological changes are common when animals are tied up or threatened or isolated from their group mates: heart rate changes and chemicals such as cortisol are released from the adrenal glands.[37] We can detect the same changes in ourselves. You are nearly knocked down by a car. You walk on, but then suddenly you feel the rush of adrenaline and notice the pounding of your heart.

Physiological measurements of body function can therefore be made using heart rate monitors and blood sampling. However, as with physiological evidence of animal feelings, these are more useful for comparisons between situations than for absolute judgements. Increased heart rate and cortisol concentration do not themselves show that a situation is stressful: indeed, animals show the same symptoms during mating. But there may be other reasons to assume that animals are stressed. When adult sows are mixed into a new group they usually fight, and they may reasonably be assumed to be stressed. John Barnett and colleagues in Australia compared different methods of mixing, and found that sows given stalls into which they could escape had lower cortisol concentrations than others. This helped them to conclude that this method was less stressful than the others.[38]

The previous section considered the minds of animals, including their feelings. This section has considered their bodies and whether they are functioning properly. Some people take a third approach to animal welfare that doesn't place so much emphasis on either minds or bodies.

Nature is wonderful

When I was growing up we had fish in a fishbowl and a pair of zebra finches in a cage. The finches were healthy and sang much of the time – although 'sang' isn't the right word for a noise described in bird books as 'like a little wooden trumpet' – but a visitor to the house once stood looking at our finches and said, 'You know, I don't think I like living things being kept in cages. It's all right for fish, and things like that, but not *living* things.' A lot of people make similar comments on the dog kept indoors all day, the poultry house with no windows, the very idea of zoos: 'It's not natural'.

The American philosopher Bernard Rollin suggests that this comes down to the idea of animal natures, which is a concept comparable to that of human nature (Box 2.3). Concern for animal welfare then poses the question 'What is necessary for animals to express their natures?' to which there have been two main answers. The first is that they must be kept in ways that allow them to perform natural behaviour. This is conveyed by Rollin's comment that 'birds gotta fly' and by the British scientist Marthe Kiley-Worthington. The second is that features of the natural environment such as sunshine and fresh air are important in themselves – a view held by the Swedish welfare campaigner Astrid Lindgren (Box 2.3).

A problem with this approach to animal welfare is that it is difficult to translate into specific recommendations or require-

---

Box 2.3   Welfare and animal natures

Bernard Rollin	Animals have natures – the pigness of the pig, the cowness of the cow, 'fish gotta swim, birds gotta fly' – which are as essential to their well-being as speech and assembly are to us.[39]
Marthe Kiley-Worthington	If we believe in evolution, then in order to avoid suffering, it is necessary over a period of time for the animal to perform all the behaviours in its repertoire.[40]
Astrid Lindgren	Let the animals see the sun just once, get away from the murderous roar of the fans. Let them get to breathe fresh air for once, instead of manure gas.[41]

ments – and most legislation is specific. Is it really necessary for a sheep to perform 'all the behaviours in its repertoire'? What about running away from wolves? Is it necessary for a hen to fly? Domestic chickens rarely fly unless they have to – and it is easy to give them an environment in which they don't have to. Is it appropriate to enshrine in law a requirement for cows to 'see the sun'?

We can't just say that animals should be kept in natural environments, for two reasons. First, natural environments are often impossible to characterize. What is the 'natural environment' of dogs, after 12 000 years of living with humans? Many other animals are also extremely adaptable: for example, rats have doubtless been living with humans, in very varied places, for a lot more than 12 000 years. Herring gulls lived on or by the sea for millennia, but many of them have now moved permanently to rubbish dumps.[42] Indeed, what is the 'natural environment' of humans?

Secondly, life in the wild is no romantic idyll. It is more often nasty, brutish and short. We tend to see animals in the wild on highly edited television programmes or on sunny days when we go for a drive in the country, and forget the cold, wet, hungry days of winter.

However, this is skirting the point. The point about respecting animal natures is not specific. It will not be addressed by drawing up another shopping list. We can respect human nature without saying what sort of house people should live in or what food they should eat, and the same goes for animals. It is not a question of whether cows specifically need to see the sun, but of treating them as cows, not as machines or humans or economic units.

It is certainly hard to translate this into practice, but progress is being made in some areas, including in the design of housing systems.[43] Some countries have also started to apply the concept of animal natures to legislation. Bernard Rollin points out that:

> Sweden has passed a law for agricultural animals that mandates that all systems of keeping farm animals must first and foremost accommodate the animals' natures. For example, the law grants cattle 'the right to graze' in perpetuity.[44]

Zoo housing of primates provides a rather different example. Gibbons are always popular in the zoo, because they spend a considerable proportion of the time hurtling acrobatically round their ropes and poles. In the wild they perform similar acrobatics in trees. It seems fair to say that it is in the nature of gibbons to climb, swing and jump, but that a well-designed climbing frame can respect this aspect of their nature about as well as branches can. The complex array of ropes, tyres, canvas and scaffolding that most zoos now provide for their lemurs, mangabeys and chimps surely allows these animals to explore, to investigate and to manipulate according to their natures, despite the absence of more easily destroyed natural materials.

Putting this approach to welfare into practice would still need a lot of work. Allowing cows to graze outdoors may solve some welfare problems but may be difficult in some countries – for example hot countries – so it would be best to identify the features of the environment that are important for animals to express their natures. Constant sunshine seems just as inappropriate for cows as constant lack of sunshine: perhaps it is variability that is important rather than sunshine as such.

Emphasis on animal natures will be particularly difficult to translate into detailed legislation. Yet it may still be useful as a corrective to the over-emphasis on specific details suggested by the other two approaches, a third leg to the animal welfare tripod of mind, body and nature.

Mind, body and nature

To recapitulate, there is a widespread consensus that we should improve animal welfare, as stressed in Chapter 1, but there is no consensus on what animal welfare is. The framework offered by David Fraser and Ian Duncan does, though, help us to clarify the concepts involved. People's views on animal welfare tend to emphasize animal feelings, animal functioning and animal nature to a greater or lesser extent: mind, body and nature (Fig. 2.4).

The three elements can actually be identified in other treatments of animal welfare. For example, the Brambell Committee, mentioned earlier, referred to both the physical and mental well-being of the animal. In addition, it said that:

> In principle we disapprove of a degree of confinement which necessarily frustrates most of the major activities which make up the animal's natural behaviour.[11]

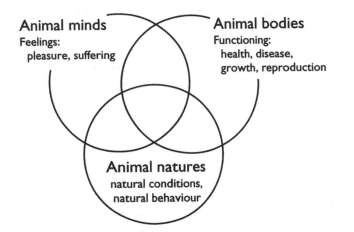

Fig. 2.4 Animal welfare: mind, body and nature. People's concepts of welfare emphasize animal minds, animal bodies, animal natures or a combination of these. The concepts overlap, but not completely.

In other words it recognized the importance of each of body, mind and nature.

Similarly, the three elements can be identified in one of the most widely quoted formulations relevant to animal welfare: the five freedoms listed by the UK's Farm Animal Welfare Council (FAWC) (Box 2.4).

Box 2.4   FAWC's Five Freedoms

Freedom from hunger and thirst	by ready access to fresh water and a diet to maintain full health and vigour
Freedom from discomfort	by providing an appropriate environment, including shelter and a comfortable resting area
Freedom from pain, injury and disease	by prevention or rapid diagnosis and treatment
Freedom to express normal behaviour	by providing sufficient space, proper facilities and company of the animal's own kind
Freedom from fear and distress	by ensuring conditions and treatment which avoid mental suffering[45]

There is sometimes confusion between FAWC's five freedoms and part of the Brambell Report, which stated that farm animals should have freedom 'to stand up, lie down, turn around, groom themselves and stretch their limbs'.[11] This list was also known as the Five Freedoms until it was largely superseded by FAWC's five freedoms.

FAWC was set up by the UK government but acts independently to advise the government and others. It suggests that the welfare of animals should be considered with reference to the five freedoms:

> These freedoms define ideal states rather than attempt to define standards for acceptable welfare. They form a logical and comprehensive framework for the analysis of welfare within any system.[45]

The list is not definitive, and there is no particular reason why it is grouped into five headings rather than four or six, but it provides a useful categorization of different factors. It will come up occasionally in this book, but it does suffer the limitations of a list approach, because the factors in the list may be contradictory. This was recognized by John Webster, an active member of FAWC closely involved in drawing up the five freedoms:

> Absolute attainment of all five freedoms is unrealistic, indeed they are to some extent incompatible. Complete behavioural freedom, for example, is unhygienic for all us animals![46]

Some of this incompatibility is because the list includes all three approaches to animal welfare: feelings (such as pain and fear), functioning (injury and disease) and naturalness or normality. Fraser and his colleagues remind us that there are disagreements between those who take the different approaches:

> Different conceptions of animal welfare can, of course, lead to conflicting conclusions about how animals ought to be treated. Observer A, favouring a functioning-based conception, may conclude that the welfare of a group of sows tethered in stalls is high because the animals are well fed, reproducing efficiently and free from disease and injury. Observer B, using a feelings-based conception, concludes that the welfare of the same animals is poor because they give vocalizations that are

thought to indicate frustration, and they escape from the stalls whenever the chance arises. Observer C, relying on a natural-living conception, agrees that the sows' welfare is poor because stalls are unnatural environments which prevent the animals' natural behaviour.[2]

Such disagreements are unavoidable. That should not be a surprise: there is no consensus on what constitutes a good life for humans either.

Nonetheless, the three approaches do overlap heavily, as suggested in Fig. 2.4. Some improvements to animal welfare are relatively uncontroversial. Astrid Lindgren said that animals should breathe fresh air rather than 'manure gas'. Few would disagree with this, because it should reduce suffering and improve functioning, as well as being more natural. Perhaps we should concentrate more on the areas of agreement and less on the areas of disagreement.

It has been worthwhile to explore issues such as anthropomorphism, and Fraser and Duncan's framework, at some length rather than just presenting a definition such as FAWC's five freedoms, because it is important to understand animal welfare rather than just taking it as read. One further, important part of understanding is the difference between different animal species. We shall go on to consider this complex issue in Chapter 3.

Conclusions

- The view that animal welfare is important is shared by most people, including nearly all scientists. This rejects the theoretical argument that animals might really be like unfeeling machines.
- It is wrong to assume that animals are like humans, although there are similarities. We must find a middle path between uncritical anthropomorphism and viewing animals as machines.
- Different concepts of welfare are possible, and different people believe one of these or a mixture. Firstly, animal welfare may concern feelings such as pleasure and suffering. Secondly, it may concern health, fitness and other aspects of functioning. Thirdly, welfare may consist of living in natural conditions. These concepts emphasize animal minds, bodies and natures, respectively.

- There are many areas of agreement between people with different concepts of welfare. However, there are also inevitably areas of disagreement.
- Where definite decisions about welfare are needed, including in legislation, a clear understanding of welfare is necessary. Such decisions will be most firmly based, and acceptable to the greatest possible number of people, if they take into account all three concepts of animal minds, bodies and natures.

References

1. Fraser, D. (1995) Science, values and animal welfare: exploring the 'inextricable connection'. *Animal Welfare*, **4**, 103–17.
2. Fraser, D., Weary, D.M., Pajor, E.A. & Milligan, B.N. (1997) A scientific conception of animal welfare that reflects ethical concerns. *Animal Welfare*, **6**, 187–205.
3. Descartes, R. (1641) From a selection reprinted under the title Animals are Machines, In *Animal Rights and Human Obligations*, 2nd edn., 1989, (eds T. Regan & P. Singer), pp. 13–9. Prentice-Hall, London.
4. Singer, P. (1975) *Animal Liberation*. New York Review of Books, New York.
5. Harrison, R. (1964) *Animal Machines: The New Factory Farming Industry*. Vincent Stuart, London.
6. Bermond, B. (1997) The myth of animal suffering. In *Animal Consciousness and Animal Ethics* (eds M. Dol, S. Kasanmoentalib, S. Lijmbach, E. Rivas & R. van den Bos), pp. 125–43. Van Gorcum, Assen, The Netherlands.
7. Kennedy, J.S. (1992) *The New Anthropomorphism*. Cambridge University Press, Cambridge.
8. Midgley, M. (1983) What is anthropomorphism? In *Animals and Why They Matter*, pp. 125–133. University of Georgia Press, Athens, Ga., USA.
9. Masson, J.M. & McCarthy, S. (1995) *When Elephants Weep: The Emotional Lives of Animals*. Delacorte, New York.
10. Skinner, B.F. (1938) *The Behavior of Animals: An Experimental Analysis*. Appleton-Century-Crofts, New York.
11. Her Majesty's Stationery Office (1965) *Report of the Technical Committee to Enquire into the Welfare of Animals kept under Intensive Livestock Husbandry Systems*. Command Paper 2836. Her Majesty's Stationery Office, London.
12. Duncan, I.J.H. & Fraser, D. (1997) Understanding animal welfare. In *Animal Welfare* (eds M.C. Appleby & B.O. Hughes), pp. 19–31. CAB International, Oxfordshire. See also ref. 2.

13. Broom, D.M. and Johnson, K.G. (1993) *Stress and Animal Welfare.* Chapman and Hall, London.
14. Oxford English Dictionary (1973, reprinted 1990) *Shorter Oxford English Dictionary.* Clarendon Press, Oxford; Chambers Dictionary (1983, reprinted 1987) *Chambers 20th Century Dictionary.* Chambers, Edinburgh.
15. Bentham, J. (1789) *Introduction to the Principles of Morals and Legislation.* 1996 Imprint. Clarendon Press, Oxford.
16. Dawkins, M.S. (1988) Behavioural deprivation: a central problem in animal welfare. *Applied Animal Behaviour Science,* **20**, 209–25.
17. Duncan, I.J.H. (1996) Animal welfare defined in terms of feelings. *Acta Agriculturae Scandinavica, Section A, Animal Science, Supplementum,* **27**, 29–35.
18. Wemelsfelder, F. (1997) Investigating the animal's point of view; an enquiry into a subject-based method of measurement in the field of animal welfare. In *Animal Consciousness and Animal Ethics* (eds M. Dol, S. Kasanmoentalib, S. Lijmbach, E. Rivas & R. van den Bos), pp. 73–89. Van Gorcum, Assen, The Netherlands.
19. See sections on hedonism and preference-fulfilment (or desire-fulfilment) in Parfit, D. (1984) *Reasons and Persons,* Appendix 1. What makes someone's life go best, pp. 493–502. Oxford University Press, Oxford.
20. Budiansky, S. (1992) *The Covenant of the Wild: Why Animals Chose Domestication.* Weidenfeld & Nicolson, London.
21. de Waal, F.B.M. (1982) *Chimpanzee Politics: Power and Sex among Apes.* Jonathan Cape, London.
22. Weary, D.M., Braithwaite, L.A. & Fraser, D. (1998) Vocal response to pain in piglets. *Applied Animal Behaviour Science,* **56**, 161–72.
23. Kent, J.E., Molony, V. & Robertson, I.S. (1995) Comparison of the Burdizzo and rubber ring methods for castrating and tail docking lambs. *Veterinary Record,* **136**, 192–6.
24. Flecknell, P.A. & Molony, V. (1997) Pain and injury. In *Animal Welfare* (eds M.C. Appleby & B.O. Hughes), pp. 63–73. CAB International, Wallingford, UK.
25. Lawrence, A.B. & Rushen, J. (eds) (1993) *Stereotypic Animal Behaviour: Fundamentals and Applications to Welfare.* CAB International, Wallingford, UK.
26. Duncan, I.J.H., Slee, G.S., Kettlewell, P., Berry, P. & Carlisle, A.J. (1986) Comparison of the stressfulness of harvesting broiler chickens by machine and by hand. *British Poultry Science,* **27**, 109–14.
27. Fraser, D. & Matthews, L.R. (1997) Preference and motivation testing. In *Animal Welfare* (eds M.C. Appleby & B.O. Hughes), pp. 159–73. CAB International, Wallingford, UK.
28. Phillips, P.A., Thompson, B.K. & Fraser, D. (1988) Preference tests of

ramp designs for young pigs. *Canadian Journal of Animal Science*, **68**, 41–8.

29. Lawrence, A.B., Appleby, M.C. & MacLeod, H.A. (1988) Measuring hunger in the pig using operant conditioning: the effect of food restriction. *Animal Production*, **47**, 131–7.

30. Appleby, M.C. & Lawrence, A.B. (1987) Food restriction as a cause of stereotypic behaviour in tethered gilts. *Animal Production*, **45**, 103–10.

31. Hughes, B.O. & Curtis, P.E. (1997) Health and disease. In *Animal Welfare* (eds M.C. Appleby & B.O. Hughes), pp. 109–25. CAB International, Wallingford, UK.

32. Broom, D.B. & Johnson, K.G. (1993) *Stress and Animal Welfare*. Chapman and Hall, London.

33. Gonyou, H.W. (1993) Animal welfare: definitions and assessment. *Journal of Agricultural and Environmental Ethics*, **6** (Suppl. 2), 37–43.

34. Broom, D.B. (1996) Animal welfare defined in terms of attempts to cope with the environment. *Acta Agriculturae Scandinavica, Section A, Animal Science, Supplementum* **27**, 22–28.

35. Curtis, S.E. (1983) *Environmental Management in Animal Agriculture*. Iowa State University Press, Ames; Wathes, C. & Charles, D. (eds) (1994) *Livestock Housing*. CAB International, Wallingford, UK.

36. Appleby, M.C., Hughes, B.O. & Elson, H.A. (1992) *Poultry Production Systems: Behaviour, Management and Welfare*. CAB International, Wallingford, UK.

37. Selye, H. (1932) The general adaptation syndrome and the diseases of adaptation. *Journal of Clinical Endocrinology*, **6**, 117–52.

38. Barnett, J.L., Cronin, G.M., McCallum, T.H., Newman, E.A. & Hennessy, D.P. (1996) Effects of grouping unfamiliar adult pigs after dark, after treatment with amperozide and by using pens with stalls, on aggression, skin lesions and plasma cortisol concentrations. *Applied Animal Behaviour Science*, **50**, 121–33.

39. Rollin, B.E. (1993) Animal production and the new social ethic for animals. In *Food Animal Well-Being* (eds B. Baumgardt & H.G. Gray), pp. 3–13. Purdue University, West Lafayette, USA.

40. Kiley-Worthington, M. (1989) Ecologicial, ethological and ethically sound environments for animals: towards symbiosis. *Journal of Agricultural Ethics*, **2**, 323–47.

41. Anonymous (1989) *How Astrid Lindgren Achieved Enactment of the 1988 Law Protecting Farm Animals in Sweden*. Animal Welfare Institute, Washington DC.

42. Furness, R.W. & Monaghan, P. (1987) *Seabird Ecology*. Blackie, Glasgow.

43. Stolba, A. & Wood-Gush, D.G.M. (1984) The identification of behavioural key features and their incorporation into a housing design for pigs. *Annales de Recherches Veterinaires*, **15**, 287–98;

Stauffacher, M. (1992) Group housing and enrichment cages for breeding, fattening and laboratory rabbits. *Animal Welfare*, **1**, 105–25.

44. Rollin, B.E. (1995) *The Frankenstein Syndrome: Ethical and Social Issues in the Genetic Engineering of Animals.* Cambridge University Press, Cambridge.

45. Farm Animal Welfare Council (1997) *Report on the Welfare of Laying Hens.* Farm Animal Welfare Council, Tolworth, UK.

46. Webster, A.J.F. (1994) *Animal Welfare: A Cool Eye Towards Eden.* Blackwell, Oxford.

Chapter 3
One big happy family: Differences between animals

Children, chimps, chickens and chiggers

Chiggers are less than a millimetre long, and they are fascinating (Fig. 3.1). They are juvenile mites, belonging to the same animal group as spiders, and if you see one under a microscope you will probably not like what you see. But when you recognize the almost incredible detail of its structure – the precisely milled jaws, the neat spiracles or holes on the side of its body for taking in air – you will marvel that something so tiny can have the organization, the complexity of body systems needed to stay alive. If you prod it with a pin or drop chemicals nearby, you will see it pull its leg in, or walk away, or writhe, or curl up and die.

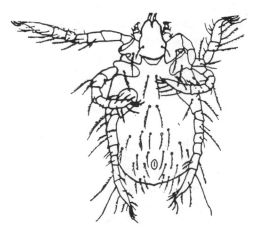

Fig. 3.1 This is a chigger – a young mite, in the same animal group as spiders – less than a millimetre long.[1] Is the welfare of such a tiny animal a valid concept?

45

When you hear that chiggers use those jaws to bite into human skin – chiggers are also known as redbugs – your initial dislike may return, but perhaps some of the fascination will remain.

Chiggers are used here as an example partly for alliteration and partly because as parasites they are more likely to prompt disgust than affection. However, the question that arises from consideration of such a tiny animal is this: is the welfare of chiggers a subject for concern? Other questions then follow. In acting to improve animal welfare, which animals matter? Which animals matter most? Does the human child matter more than the chimp, the chimp more than the chicken, the chicken more than the chigger? We will consider these questions first in relation to animal minds, then later in relation to animal bodies and animal natures.

Sentience and consciousness

The idea that welfare concerns the feelings of animals needs some development, because 'feelings' may mean either just sensations such as touch and sight or more complex processes such as pain and emotions.[2] This raises a problem, because whereas all animals, including chiggers, have at least some of the five senses, it is less clear that all animals are capable of suffering or experiencing pleasure. Can a chigger suffer?

Another word that is often used in this context is *sentience*, and some people conclude from consideration of sentience that the welfare of humans, chimps and chickens is a matter for concern but that the welfare of chiggers is not. Ian Duncan, for example, was quoted in Chapter 2 saying that 'welfare is a term which cannot be applied sensibly to the lower animals or to plants but only to sentient animals'.[3] 'Lower animals' here would certainly include mites.

However, 'sentient' has the same spread of meanings as 'feelings'. Philosopher Michael Leahy says that, 'To be sentient is to have the power of sense-perception; to see, hear, smell, taste or touch'.[4] In this sense all animals are sentient. But the term may also be used to mean 'capacity for suffering or enjoyment'.[5] It was in this sense that Duncan seems to have intended it, and this conveys the idea that some animals are capable of suffering while others are not.

Resolution of this confusion comes from the fact that there is no rigid dividing line between 'haves' and 'have nots', between animals with certain capabilities and those without. Firstly, there is no sharp distinction between sensations such as touch and feelings such as pain. Secondly, all animals have mechanisms for responding to damage or avoiding potential damage. In vertebrates these are similar to our own,[6] but the way in which the incoming messages are processed in the brain differs between species: both chimps and chickens feel pain, but in different ways. Invertebrates are more different, and there is of course huge variety among the invertebrates. Nevertheless, it makes more sense to think of feelings such as pain being present to a greater or lesser extent in different species than of them being simply present or absent. Thirdly, suffering is affected by thinking, and types of thinking vary between species. A particular animal species will therefore be able to suffer in certain ways but not others: chickens probably feel pain but not grief.

So we can say that all animals are sentient, but to varying degrees. The European Union has recently taken this approach, in declaring animals – without exclusions – to be 'sentient beings'.[7] This suggests that welfare is a matter for concern in all animals, but that what this means in practice will depend on the sentient development of particular species – and indeed particular individuals. This point will be explored further below, but it may mean that in practical terms Ian Duncan is right, that the concept of welfare has little application to relatively simple animals such as chiggers.

There is one line of argument that goes further and concludes that welfare is a matter for concern in humans and chimps but not in either chickens or chiggers. This is a sophisticated variant of the 'animals are machines' argument discussed in Chapter 2, but it is no more persuasive, as we shall see. It is based on the idea that suffering requires a highly-developed *consciousness*. Psychologist Bob Bermond has written a provocative essay called *The myth of animal suffering*.[8] He asks:

> Are animals capable of experiencing negative emotions? In posing this question, we must not forget that pain and suffering are conscious experiences. After all, it would be nonsensical to talk of experiences if those experiences failed to reach the domain of consciousness. The question regarding suffering in animals, therefore, primarily addresses the issue of whether animals have a consciousness.

Furthermore, Bermond thinks that very few animals can be said to be conscious. He reviews experimental evidence and details of brain structure, and considers that only apes and possibly dolphins are conscious. As a result he says that:

> It is concluded that emotional experiences of animals, and therefore suffering, may only be expected in anthropoid apes and possibly dolphins.

What is it, though, that humans or apes or dolphins are conscious *of*? What are they thinking *about*? They are thinking about the pain or the pleasure or the frustration. Surely they must feel pain if they are to think about feeling pain? If you burn your hand, the first thing that goes through your head is simply 'Ow!' Only afterwards do you think 'That hurt'. We are notoriously poor at knowing what is going on in our minds, so this account of human thoughts does not demonstrate the actual processes involved, but it does emphasize that feeling and thinking may be distinct.

Most people believe that many animals – such as chickens – can feel 'Ow!' without the ability to think 'That hurt' (Fig. 3.2). Part of the confusion is because consciousness is another term used with a variety of meanings. One of those meanings is 'the ability of an individual to perceive its own mental life'.[9] This is the sense used by Bermond, but is more often called self-consciousness (or self-awareness). It conveys the idea that animals have a 'sense of self', some understanding of their own existence as individuals. The most important way of investigating this has been to ask whether an animal can learn to recognize itself in a mirror. Chimps seem to be quite good at doing this but other animals are not.[10] Most people would agree that self-consciousness occurs, if at all, only in apes. Dolphins have been less investigated but are another possible special case.

Most people use the term consciousness with a broader meaning: 'awareness of the environment, sentience'.[9] Veterinarian Marc Bracke criticized the sort of definition used by Bermond. He pointed out that it would be nonsense for him to tell his client 'Madam, the anaesthetic is wearing off and your cat is returning to non-consciousness'.[11]

The resolution of this linguistic confusion is the same as for that over sentience. It makes more sense to consider consciousness not as all-or-nothing, but as something that animals may possess to a greater or lesser extent.

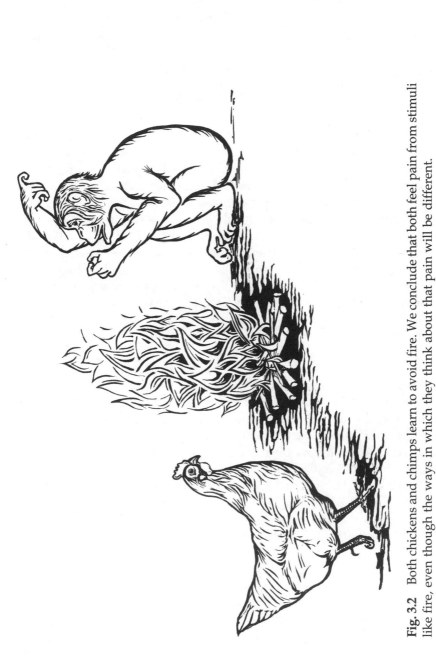

Fig. 3.2 Both chickens and chimps learn to avoid fire. We conclude that both feel pain from stimuli like fire, even though the ways in which they think about that pain will be different.

So again we conclude that suffering occurs to a greater or lesser extent in different species, and that different species may experience different kinds of suffering, but that it is not productive to attempt any categorization of animals into those that can suffer and those that cannot.

All animals are equal ...

The fact that there is variation between species in the extent and nature of their feelings is not surprising. We must now move on to our second kind of question and decide, given this variation, what priority should be given to the welfare of different species.

Some people would say, if asked, that the welfare of a human matters more than that of a chimp, and the welfare of a chimp more than that of a chicken. Is this justified? One possibility is that this belief gives too much emphasis to animal feelings – to animal minds. The complementary emphases on animal bodies and animal natures outlined in Chapter 2 give a different picture, and this issue will be considered shortly. First, though, it is necessary to explore further the implications of animal feelings for animal welfare.

Thinking affects suffering, as already mentioned. A chimp may indeed think about pain, and suffer more as a result. A human may worry so much about whether a pain means something serious that it comes to dominate life. But conversely a human may understand that a pain is temporary, or even that it is necessary for longer-term welfare. 'I'm sorry,' says the doctor, 'this injection will be rather sore, but you should feel better by tomorrow.' The fact that highly developed cognition may reduce suffering in some instances, rather than increase it, was appreciated nearly 2000 years ago by Lucius Columella of Rome, who wrote a treatise on agriculture in the first century:

> The delivery of a pregnant ewe should be watched over with as much care as midwives exercise; for this animal produces its offspring just in the same way as a woman, and its labour is painful even more often since it is devoid of all reasoning.[12]

The point is that while a reasoning human may suffer more than a sheep in some circumstances, the human may suffer less in others. There is no simple correlation between brain power and suffering, and the same amount of suffering matters to the sheep just as much as it does to the human. There will certainly be times when we could say that a ewe is suffering as much as she possibly could – that she is suffering 100%, so to speak. At such times, who is to say that her suffering matters less than a human's? A particular human may well think that the sheep's suffering matters less than their own, but that is a separate issue, to which we shall also return shortly. The welfare of an animal matters to that animal just as much as your welfare matters to you.

Suppose that a neutral observer – a compassionate Martian, for example – has to adjudicate between a woman and a ewe who are both in pain (Fig. 3.3). The Martian has one dose of painkiller. There are circumstances in which he might give it to the woman: perhaps she asks for it and he understands her language, whereas the ewe remains silent. There are circumstances in which he might give it to the ewe: he has read Columella's treatise (in the original Latin) and pities her unreasoning fear. But these circumstances are incidental – there is no fundamental reason why he should favour either the human or the sheep.

This sort of argument has been widely used, as here, to compare suffering in animals and humans. Peter Singer, for example,

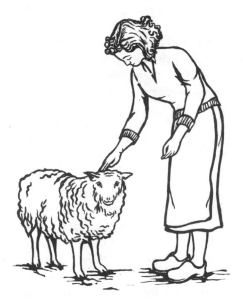

Fig. 3.3   If a woman and a ewe are both in pain, which should receive priority? A neutral judge would say neither.

criticizes the assumption that suffering in humans is more important than that in animals.[5] As we saw in Chapter 1, he says that this assumption is speciesist, an unreasonable bias in favour of the species to which we happen to belong. The same argument obviously applies to comparisons between different animal species. It implies that the welfare of a chimp does not matter more than that of a chicken.

The general conclusion is that there should be *equal consideration of similar interests*, regardless of what species has those interests. That sounds radical, and there are some dissenters,[13] but it is perhaps not as radical as it sounds. Here is one example of it being put into practice. Until recently, anyone doing an animal experiment in Denmark was required by law to use 'lower' animals rather than 'higher' whenever possible. The meaning of 'lower' and 'higher' wasn't even based on any principle such as brain power: the law meant that mice or rats should be used rather than, say, dogs. The Danish Ethical Council for Animals concluded that this was unjustified.[14] Why should the suffering of a mouse matter less than that of a dog? Danish law has been changed, and the expectation is now that if an experiment is necessary it will be done on the species most appropriate for achieving its aims – which might mean, for example, that it could be done on a small number of dogs rather than a large number of mice.

One reason why 'equal consideration' sounds radical is that it sounds as if it puts all animals on an equal footing. What about chiggers? Well, writers who emphasize equal consideration, such as Singer, relate it to sentience. Singer says that:

> The capacity for suffering and enjoyment is a prerequisite for having interests at all, a condition that must be satisfied before we can speak of interests in a meaningful way.[5]

The capacity of chiggers for suffering and enjoyment is very different from that of species with more highly developed sentience – different, and in at least some ways more limited. So just as we said that in practice Ian Duncan is right, that the concept of welfare has little application to simple animals like chiggers, we can agree with Singer that in practice it is not meaningful to speak of chiggers as having interests. To reiterate the more general point, that does not mean that there is a list of animals with interests and another list without – there is a continuum across species in the extent to which they have interests.

One other reason why 'equal consideration of similar interests' is not as radical as it first appears is that interests also vary in other ways between species, as we shall see in the next section.

... But some animals are more equal than others

Even if the welfare of humans, chimps and chickens is of equal importance, that does not mean that it is identical in nature. The welfare of different species is affected in different ways by the environment, and safeguarded by different conditions. To come straight to the point, humans are more complex than chimps, and chimps than chickens. They are more developed in many characteristics, such as rationality, sociality, self-awareness and autonomy.[15] So a human has interests that a chimp doesn't – such as reading or listening to stories. And a chimp has interests that a chicken doesn't – such as living with her mother for many years.[16] 'Equal consideration of similar interests' sounds radical partly because writers like Singer have emphasized certain interests that are similar between different species – such as not being in pain. Where species have dissimilar interests they may be treated differently. They should be treated differently.

The welfare of humans needs much more complex conditions to safeguard it than does the welfare of chimps and chickens. Similarly, if we have both chimps and chickens under our care, we need to give much more attention to the welfare of the former than the latter. Chimps need a richer, more varied environment than chickens, and a social group that is stable for years rather than months, if their interests are to be fully taken into account (Fig. 3.4).

We reach a similar conclusion if we stop considering just animal interests, or animal feelings, and consider also how to safeguard the functioning of animal bodies or the expression of animal natures. A young chimpanzee has many more requirements for proper growth and development than a chick does. In the wild he needs to get his mother's milk. He needs to learn how to use tools. If he is to survive and to reproduce, he needs to learn social skills in the group. So if we are looking after him, we should give him the opportunities to do all these things, or satisfactory substitutes.

An emphasis on animal bodies and animal natures also

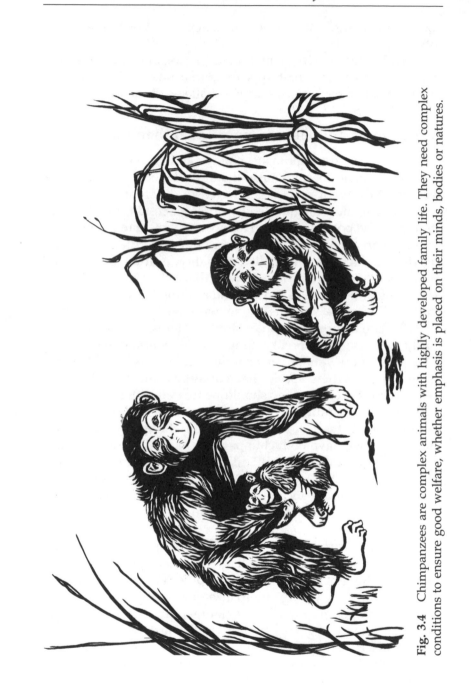

Fig. 3.4 Chimpanzees are complex animals with highly developed family life. They need complex conditions to ensure good welfare, whether emphasis is placed on their minds, bodies or natures.

reinforces the point that concern for welfare is not all-or-nothing. Different species have more or less complex minds, bodies and natures, so they need more or less complex conditions to safeguard their welfare.

We cannot go as far as saying that we must always safeguard animal minds, bodies *and* natures, because we saw in Chapter 2 that the implications of these concepts may be contradictory, but perhaps we can say that we should *consider* animal minds, bodies and natures, as and when appropriate. In the present context, this approach means that it is appropriate to consider the welfare of species with relatively simple development of sentience, in at least some circumstances. The welfare of chiggers is not a contradiction in terms. Biologists Henk Verhoog and Thijs Visser have suggested that we overemphasize the importance of consciousness for welfare because we humans are conscious. They say that it is being alive that is important: we should give moral consideration to all living things. Thereafter they take a similar approach to the one we have reached here: different living things differ in their natures and their needs, and we should take account of this in how we treat them.[17]

Are we back where we started? Do humans matter more than chimps, more than chickens, more than chiggers? The answer is no, for three reasons. Firstly, the idea that the welfare of one species – particularly humans – is more important than that of another is really the wrong way of looking at things: it is of equal importance to the individuals concerned.

Secondly, the principle that similar interests deserve equal consideration is well grounded, and has important implications. Animals do not have all the same interests as humans, but they do have some interests in common – like avoiding pain and hunger. Many people recognize this with regard to their pets. In Chapter 2 we talked about someone living alone with a dog. That man would share his last crust with his animal companion. Such an attitude contrasts strikingly with that of people who think that all medical experiments on animals are justified.

Thirdly, while complexity is one factor that affects how we should treat animals, with more complex animals having more complex requirements to achieve comparable welfare, it is not the only factor. In the next section these factors will be explored, to establish how we actually sort out our priorities in the treatment of animals.

First, second and third among equals

Suppose we call in our neutral observer again, our friendly Martian. He has decided that the welfare of all species matters equally. He accepts, though, that more effort needs to be allocated to looking after complex species than simple ones. What other factors affect his judgement on priorities?

One possible factor is rarity. The Martian might feel that it is more important to look after individuals of a rare species than a common one. However, this is not so much a question of welfare as of survival: the motivation for looking after rare animals is to prevent them going extinct, not because they need any more care as individuals. This issue will be covered in the next chapter.

There is one other major factor. Our neutral Martian isn't allocating his own effort, isn't spending his own money. If he was, he wouldn't be neutral. The other major questions are: who is making the decisions; whose effort is being allocated; whose time, or energy, or money is involved? Maybe it is a woman who has to decide whether to feed her sheep or a starving dog. Maybe it is a man who has to decide whether to feed his dog or a starving sheep. Either way, the Martian will not expect those people to be as neutral as he is himself, but nor will he expect them to be completely self-centred.

Ethical arguments do not generally tell us that we should be completely neutral, unselfish or impartial. Those that do, such as a strict interpretation of utilitarianism, are unreasonably demanding,[18] and it was pointed out in Chapter 1 that few people are pure utilitarians. What most ethical arguments do is to remind us that we shouldn't be completely selfish or partial. They do not tell us exactly where the right balance lies between unselfishness and selfishness, although they may help us in finding that balance. One message of this book is that humans have been too selfish in their dealings with animals and should be more fair to animals in future: that is another way of phrasing the argument that we should do more for animal welfare.

The message of this section is that in allocating our efforts between different species and individual animals, we have been too strongly influenced by our own preferences – to an extent that can be described as selfish or unfair. It is understandable and reasonable that we are influenced by our own needs, our own preferences, and some of these needs and preferences are explored in Box 3.1. This is another part of Mary Midgley's

---

Box 3.1   Concern for different categories of animals

People are more concerned for the welfare of some types of animals than others. Here are some of the factors that affect this:

Usefulness/ inconvenience	Useful animals may be either favoured or regarded with indifference, while the welfare of inconvenient animals such as parasites is rarely a matter of concern.
Likeness to ourselves	Primates, furry mammals, birds that are also warm blooded, may all be preferred to more alien species.
Attractiveness	Some species very different from ourselves, like butterflies, are seen as attractive.
Size	Large animals are often flavoured over small ones.
Visibility	If rats came out of their holes when poisoned, people would be more concerned. They know poisoned rats die slowly but are able to ignore this.
Rarity	Unusual animals are more interesting. Even preferred animals may fall out of favour if too common, like stray cats and dogs.
Companionship	Even an insect may be treated as a companion.
Familiarity	Our attitude to animals is affected by experience, including how they are presented in books and on television.[19]

---

argument, presented in Chapter 1, that it is understandable and reasonable that we favour those near to us. It is understandable and reasonable that one person favours her sheep over a dog and that another favours his dog over a sheep. However, we have too readily favoured bright and beautiful animals over others that are merely useful, whose needs are just as great.

Here is one clear example. In many countries it is illegal to keep birds in cages that are too small for them to stretch their wings. Any birds, that is, except poultry. Poultry are specifically excluded from these laws[20] and chickens can be kept in battery cages. Now suppose that you have a canary in a cage (as discussed in Chapter 2) and you also keep chickens. You are not expected to be completely neutral between the two. You keep the canary in your living room for her beauty and companionship, and it is acceptable that you should give her better conditions and more care than your chickens. Yet our Martian judge would surely find it unreasonable that you are allowed to keep your chickens in cages so small that they cannot stretch their wings, just because you are keeping them for economic reasons rather than for pleasure (and larger cages cost more). He would surely judge that to be unfair. It isn't necessarily you that is being unfair, but humans are certainly being unfair at the expense of chickens. Society is being unfair in the distinction it makes between canaries and chickens, in its allocation of effort, its legislation to safeguard the welfare of one more than the other. We do not expect completely equal treatment of the similar interests of canaries and chickens, but fairness demands more similar treatment in the future than in the past.

The same arguments apply to the ways in which we treat different individual animals of the same species. The fact that we keep pet mice in large, comfortable cages while poisoning mice in the kitchen has often been pointed out. D.S. Favre, Professor of Law in Detroit, tells the story of four rabbits, with acknowledgements to Beatrix Potter. His story is abbreviated here:

> While everyone knows of the adventures of Peter Rabbit and his sisters, not everyone knows of what happened later in their lives. The next summer, Mr McGregor set out half a dozen box traps, and as fate would have it, Flopsy, Mopsy and Cottontail were all caught in the traps. Flopsy was sold as a pet. Mopsy was bought by the local zoo. Cottontail was purchased by a company which sold rabbits to scientific research facilities and universities.
>
> Mr McGregor's neighbour, Mr Jones, decided to attempt the same. The next day he set out some steel jaw traps as the first step in making fur lined gloves.[21]

We can imagine that the subsequent welfare of Flopsy, Mopsy

and Cottontail was very different, not to mention that of their other brothers and sisters who fell prey to Mr Jones. Favre comments that the laws governing different uses of rabbits vary widely, and also differ considerably between different countries. He concludes that this is inappropriate:

> If we are willing to admit that a rabbit is a rabbit regardless of who owns it or where it is being held, then it is apparent that only one set of standards is necessary to protect rabbits around the world.

True, although again it is a question of finding the right balance. We don't expect Mr Jones to treat his daughter's pet rabbit and the rabbit in his vegetable garden in the same way, but we can ask that he doesn't use steel jaw traps or slow-acting poison for the latter.

It is also important to remember that people differ in their needs and preferences. Some need companionship and are particularly concerned to improve the welfare of pets. Some disapprove of pet keeping and campaign for better treatment of wildlife. To some extent these various needs and preferences, favouring different categories of animal, will themselves result in a balanced outcome. If Mr McGregor disapproves of steel jaw traps he may influence Mr Jones. If Mr Jones dislikes zoos he may discourage Mr McGregor from selling any more rabbits there. Politicians tend to respond to the most active lobbies in drawing up legislation, and there are lobbies acting as proponents for many categories of animals. However, this will not be a complete balance, partly because not every category of animals has its proponents, and partly because there are lobbies for other interests. Those people who lobby for farm animal welfare, for example, are opposed by those who lobby for cheaper food production.

The position we have reached is as follows. The welfare of all animals should be considered, and the welfare of all species – or at least all those with more than minimal sentience – is of equal importance to the individuals concerned. So for complete fairness there should be equal consideration of similar interests. More complex animals have more complex interests, so they need more complex conditions to achieve similar welfare and more effort to care for them if they are under human responsibility. In fact, people have tended to allocate their effort to animals, and between different species and individual animals, according to their own, human needs and preferences. To some extent this is reasonable because nobody can be expected to be completely neutral and unselfish. However, it has been taken to an unreasonable extent, and a better balance needs to be achieved between human needs, the needs of all animals, and the needs of particular categories of animals.

One big happier family

Certain aspects of the better balance between human and animal needs will cost time, energy and money. Some people still jib at this. 'Resources are limited,' they say. 'There is only so much room in the lifeboat.' However, Mary Midgley turns this lifeboat model round to give us a picture that is more reminiscent of Noah's Ark:

> The problem of competition presents itself to many people in a form more or less like this: Must we really acknowledge all our long-lost cousins and heave them into the humanitarian life-boat, which is already foundering under the human race? Or can we take another look at the rule-book and declare the relationship too distant, so that we are justified in letting the whole lot sink?
> The two solutions just mentioned are, however, extreme views, programmes of absolute dismissal and absolute inclusion. The point is that we are not usually in lifeboats. I am tempted to say that life is never like this. A recent Oxfam pamphlet answered lifeboat-style objections to international aid by remarking that 10% of the world's population now consumes 90% of its resources. Whatever sort of a situation that may be, it does not seem to be a lifeboat one for the 10%. In the end, we are all in the same boat.[22]

Peter Sandøe and his colleagues make a similar point explicitly with regard to care of farm animals:

> Broiler chickens, stalled sows and other farm animals will often suffer and will lack the ability to do things which could contribute to their 'positive welfare'. The interests of these animals are set aside so that production can be efficient and that consumers can buy cheap meat and other animal

products. However, in the rich part of the world these cheap products are not vital to human interests. If we paid 30 or 50% more and the extra money was used to improve the living conditions of the animals this would mean an immense increase in their welfare. In a country like Denmark where ordinary consumers spend less than 13% of their available income on food this would have only a marginal effect on income available for other purposes, and since income is generally high it would not significantly decrease the welfare of the affected humans. Therefore according to the utilitarian view we ought to make radical changes in the way farm animals are being treated.[23]

Their point is particularly striking if we contrast the treatment of farm animals with that of pets (like the canary discussed above), on which a considerable amount of money is spent. Most of us could afford to treat animals better, and could afford more fairness in how we treat different categories of animals.

Furthermore, other aspects of the better balance will not cost any time, energy or money. They will just require a change of attitude. As an illustration, here is an account from the magazine *Deer*, which mostly deals with shooting. The author was sitting in a high-seat at twilight:

> I heard a desperate squeaking noise and was convinced that a fox had caught a roe deer kid. As I peered into the growing darkness the fox ran out onto the track carrying something in its mouth. By now it was barely visible. Leaning over and looking through the telescopic sight I momentarily saw the fox and fired hoping that at best I had managed to kill it but if not, that at least it had dropped the roe kid as it was at least 75 metres away.
>
> When I reached the spot, to my amazement and as I had hoped, the fox was lying dead. The fawn was sitting quietly in between its mouth and front legs completely unharmed.[24]

The author was concerned for the welfare of a roe kid (which is ironic considering that he was there to shoot adult roe deer) but oblivious to the risk of injury and suffering for the fox. A change of attitude to recognize the importance of welfare in different categories of animals would cost him nothing. Perhaps he has already had such a change of attitude since the article appeared in 1980, but perhaps not.

The eighteenth century poet William Cowper made a similar point when he stressed that inhumane behaviour is often unnecessary:

> I would not enter on my list of friends
> (Tho' grac'd with polish'd manners and fine sense,
> Yet wanting sensibility) the man
> Who needlessly sets foot upon a worm.[25]

In this instance the suffering of the worm was restricted, both because the sentience of worms is relatively simple and because it died quickly. However, the description of 'inhumane behaviour' still seems to apply. This raises the question of how attitudes to animal welfare are related to attitudes to killing animals, a question that will be addressed in Chapter 4.

Conclusions

- Mental processes relevant to welfare – especially feelings, sentience and consciousness – are not all-or-nothing. All animals are sentient to varying degrees.
- More complex animals have more complex interests, so they need more effort to care for them if they are under human responsibility. The same applies if we are to safeguard the functioning of animal bodies or the expression of animal natures.
- For complete fairness there should be equal consideration of similar interests, but people have allocated priorities according to their own, human needs and preferences.
- A better balance needs to be achieved between human needs, the needs of all animals, and the needs of particular categories of animals.

References

1. Figure from Ruppert, E.E. & Barnes, R.D. (1994) *Invertebrate Zoology*, 6th edn. Saunders, Philadelphia.
2. Chambers Dictionary (1983, reprinted 1987) *Chambers 20th Century Dictionary*. Chambers, Edinburgh.
3. Duncan, I.J.H. (1996) Animal welfare defined in terms of feelings. *Acta Agriculturae Scandinavica, Section A, Animal Science, Supplementum* **27**, 29–35.

4. Leahy, M.P.T. (1991) *Against Liberation: Putting Animals in Perspective.* Routledge, London.

5. Singer, P. (1975) *Animal Liberation.* New York Review of Books, New York.

6. Gentle, M.J. (1997) Acute and chronic pain in the chicken. In *Proceedings, 5th European Symposium on Poultry Welfare* (eds P. Koene & H.J. Blokhuis), pp. 5–11; Kestin, S.C. (1994) *Pain and Stress in Fish.* RSPCA, Horsham, Sussex.

7. UK Ministry of Agriculture, Fisheries and Food (1997) News release. 18th June.

8. Bermond, B. (1997) The myth of animal suffering. In *Animal Consciousness and Animal Ethics* (eds M. Dol, S. Kasanmoentalib, S. Lijmbach, E. Rivas & R. van den Bos), pp. 125–43. Van Gorcum, Assen, The Netherlands.

9. Walker, P.M.B. (1988) *Chambers Science and Technology Dictionary.* Chambers, Cambridge.

10. Gallup, G.G. (1979) Self-awareness in primates. *American Scientist,* **67**, 417–21; Heyes, C.M. (1994) Reflections on self-recognition in primates. *Animal Behaviour,* **47**, 909–19.

11. Marc Bracke's comment was made at a conference, Perspectives on Animal Consciousness, at Wageningen, The Netherlands, July 1997.

12. Forster, E.S. & Heffner, E.H. (trans.) (1968) *Lucius Junius Moderatus Columella on Agriculture, vol. II, Loeb Classical Library 407.* Heinemann, London.

13. Carruthers, P. (1992) *The Animals Issue: Moral Theory in Practice.* Cambridge University Press, Cambridge.

14. Professor Peter Sandøe, Chair, Danish Ethical Council for Animals, personal communication.

15. DeGrazia, D. (1996) *Taking Animals Seriously: Mental Life and Moral Status.* Cambridge University Press, Cambridge.

16. Goodall, J. (1986) *The Chimpanzees of Gombe: Patterns of Behaviour.* Harvard University Press, Cambridge, MA.

17. Verhoog, H. & Visser, T. (1997) A view of intrinsic value not based on animal consciousness. In *Animal Consciousness and Animal Ethics* (eds M. Dol, S. Kasanmoentalib, S. Lijmbach, E. Rivas & R. van den Bos), pp. 223–32. Van Gorcum, Assen, The Netherlands.

18. Williams, B. (1972) *Morality: An Introduction to Ethics.* Cambridge University Press, Cambridge.

19. Paul, L. (1993) Pet ownership in childhood: its influence on attitudes towards animals. *Applied Animal Behaviour Science,* **35**, 296.

20. Brooman, S. & Legge, D. (1997) *Law Relating to Animals.* Cavendish, London.

21. Favre, D.S. (1989) Movement towards an international convention for the protection of animals – the further adventures of four rabbits. In *Animal Welfare and the Law* (eds D.E. Blackman, P.N. Hum-

phreys & P. Todd), pp. 247–70. Cambridge University Press, Cambridge.

22. Midgley, M. (1983) *Animals and Why They Matter*. University of Georgia Press, Athens, Ga., USA. (The quotation is abbreviated.)
23. Sandøe, P., Crisp, R. & Holtug, N. (1997) Ethics. In *Animal Welfare* (eds M.C. Appleby & B.O. Hughes), pp. 3–17. CAB International, Wallingford, UK.
24. Langmead, M.J. (1980) Saving a roe kid from a fox. *Deer*, **5**, 30–31.
25. Cowper, W. (1788) The winter walk at noon. *Poems*, 4th edn. Book 6, p. 560. Johnson, London.

Chapter 4
To have and to hold:
Keeping and killing animals

Use and abuse

We have been talking about improvement of animal welfare. However, much of the rhetoric about animal treatment and protection, in street demonstrations and in the media, takes a different approach. Ban cosmetic testing on animals, it says. Stop eating meat. Close down zoos and circuses. This rhetoric implies that we can't use animals without abusing them. Further, it implies that much use of animals is, unavoidably, abuse. So we shouldn't use them.

This sort of approach often has a logical basis. For example, if you believe in animal rights and that animals have a right not to be killed for our convenience, then it is logical to argue that we shouldn't keep and kill animals for food. However, we saw in Chapter 1 that it is difficult to carry such logic through and to accept all its conclusions. The theory of animal rights provides a framework, but leaves us with many difficult decisions to make. Similarly, utilitarianism is persuasive within limits; it is less so when taken to extremes, and few people are pure utilitarians.

This chapter examines the implications of our use and abuse of animals, the question of whether we could stop using them, set them free, leave them alone, and the effects that this would have. The chapter concentrates on those animals that we do use, but some of the discussion is also relevant to our interactions with other animals, such as parasites, pests and wildlife.

To begin with, the very concept of use of animals involves a major assumption: that the relationship is not just asymmetrical but wholly one-sided. We are using animals. They are being used by us. Our interests are being served. Theirs are not. In fact, this is never the whole truth. Whatever the use we make of animals, they do receive some benefit. They receive food and shelter. In many cases they receive life. We may well be in control, and may well receive the lion's share of the rewards to be gained, but there is mutual benefit involved in almost every case. This suggests that it is helpful to think about the interactions between humans and animals – and about how these interactions should be made more fair to both parties – rather than just about human use of animals.

This argument is a double-edged sword. It removes some of the strength from criticism of human use and abuse of animals. However, it also emphasizes that the relationship is two-sided, and that since we are indeed in control it is our responsibility to look after both sides, not just our own.

The two-sided nature of the relationship is sometimes expressed in terms of an implicit contract between humans and animals. They help us, so we look after them. American science writer Stephen Budiansky[1] has gone further in relation to domestic animals and refers to 'the covenant of the wild'. This is a development of an idea from Raymond Coppinger,[2] that the ancestors of our domestic animals played an active part in forming relationships with humans. Those relationships became mutually beneficial, and still remain so. Coppinger and Budiansky say that animals chose domestication, rather than having it forced upon them. This is partly true for dogs: it is likely that the relationship between humans and dogs began with dogs scavenging from humans rather than humans capturing dogs.[3] It is probably not literally true for other species, such as sheep, goats and cattle. However, there is a sense in which it is useful to think of the ancestors of domestic species as having made an appropriate 'choice'. This is because their descendants have been much more successful – at least in terms of numbers – than other individuals of the same species that remained wild. There are 1.3 billion cattle in the world.[4] Domestic horses are widespread, whereas wild horses have almost died out. Chickens are by far the most numerous birds on earth.

Similar arguments also apply to other animals that we keep – to pets, zoo animals and laboratory animals. Some species of animal only occur in captivity. Père David's deer, for example, were extinct in the wild for many years: they only existed in zoos (Fig. 4.1). All these animals gain from their relationship with us.

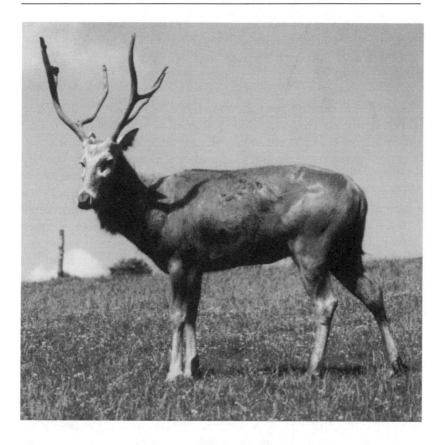

Fig. 4.1 Père David's Deer were discovered in a park in China by a missionary of that name. They existed nowhere else, but they are now in zoos worldwide and some have recently been released into the wild.[5]

Which is not to say, of course, that they gain as much as they should.

Whose life is it anyway?

We are certainly in control. Budiansky[1] speaks of 'the perpetual problem that nature has posed for us in managing the inevitably conflicting interests of earth's inhabitants'. John Webster,

Professor of Animal Husbandry at Bristol University, talks of man's dominion over animals. This phrase is a quotation from Robert Burns' poem *To a mouse*, and Burns in turn was quoting from the Bible.

> Man has dominion over the animals whether we like it or not. Wherever we share space on the planet, and this includes all but the most inaccessible regions of land, sea and air, it is we not they that determine where and how they will live. We may elect to put hens in a battery cage or establish a game reserve to preserve the tiger but in each case the decision is ours, not theirs ... We admire the tiger not only for its fearful symmetry but as a symbol of freedom itself, so we offer it rather more freedom than we would think fit for the chicken. It is impossible, however, to avoid the issue that both the chicken and the tiger are living on our terms.[6]

One issue that comes up here concerning animals which we keep is the question of ownership. We referred in earlier chapters to a man and his dog, to a farmer and his cows (Fig. 4.2) , to a woman and her sheep. In what sense do we 'own' sentient creatures? Some people have become very sensitive to this issue, which is one reason for introduction of the term 'companion animal' instead of 'pet', because it seems to carry less connotation of ownership. Such people sometimes talk about 'the dog who lives with me' to avoid using the phrase 'my dog'.

To some extent this is a red herring. The words 'his', 'her', 'my' and so on are not as important as they may appear. They may seem to put the animals on a par with inanimate objects, to suggest an equivalence between 'my cow' and 'my cow shed', between 'my cat' and 'my bicycle'. However, we also use the same words in other contexts: we talk about 'my country' and 'my mother' – about 'Noah and his sons'. It is how we treat the animals that matters, not the language we use about them. Ben may tell everyone that his dog is a stupid good-for-nothing, but if he treats her well she isn't to know.

On the other hand, language can affect our attitude to animals – and hence our treatment of them. The character in Dostoevsky's *Crime and Punishment* who beats a horse to death obviously has the attitude that she is his horse, to do with as he likes. That attitude might well be influenced by the language of possession: 'She's mine, after all. What's it got to do with you?'

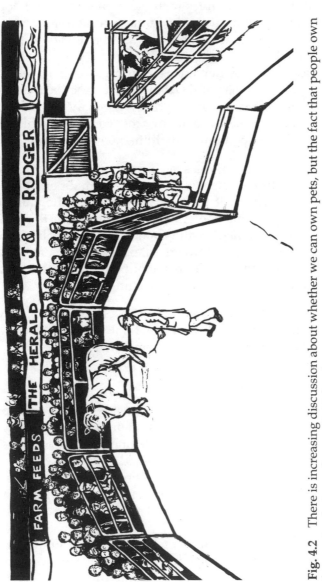

Fig. 4.2 There is increasing discussion about whether we can own pets, but the fact that people own farm animals is rarely questioned.

The animal trainer Vicki Hearne has discussed at some length the question of how we talk about animals.[7] For example, it has been common to refer to animals as 'it' rather than 'he' or 'she', to talk about 'the dog that lives with me' rather than 'the dog who lives with me', to put inverted commas round animal names, as in the dog called 'Lassie'. Suffice it to say that this book generally avoids these things.

The question of ownership is also important in legislation. Indeed, Simon Brooman and Debbie Legge describe the property status of animals as a 'contemporary anomaly' in English law (and it is similar in the law of many other countries) which affects even animals we don't normally think about owning:

> The treatment of animals as property without rights is a common feature of the law relating to animals: an abuse of an animal is an abuse of the human interest in the animal concerned; over-fishing the Atlantic fish stocks is the loss of a public environmental resource; poaching results in the loss of possible financial gain through sale; the hunting of a species to near extinction raises concerns about the loss of rare species to be enjoyed by future generations, and so on.[8]

Legislation will be discussed further in Chapter 9. For now, we will note again that it is how we treat animals that matters, whether they belong to us or to themselves.

A life worth living

So because of our control, our influence – and perhaps our ownership – there are many cows, many chickens, many pets, many laboratory animals in the world and we have to address the issue of whether this is to be welcomed.

Perhaps the key question here, but one that is rarely addressed, is whether the life of a cow, a chicken, a pet or a laboratory animal is worth living. It is not as good as it could be, but is it better than never having been born at all?

Let us address this question first in relation to animals' minds, or feelings. We can give considerable substance to this question if we assume, with Tom Regan, that animals think and feel in ways similar to ourselves:

> We are each of us the experiencing subject of a life, a conscious creature having an individual welfare that has importance to

us whatever our usefulness to others. We want and prefer things, believe and feel things, recall and expect things. And all these dimensions of our life, including our pleasure and pain, our enjoyment and suffering, our satisfaction and frustration, our continued existence or our untimely death – all make a difference to the quality of our life as lived, as experienced, by us as individuals. As the same is true of those animals that concern us (the ones that are eaten and trapped, for example), they too must be viewed as the experiencing subjects of a life.[9]

Even if we don't agree with Regan's assumptions, we can consider the good and bad things that happen to an animal (affecting its mind, its body or its nature) adding up over time. Henrik Simonsen, a Danish vet, has given us a pictorial image of this (Fig. 4.3). Now Simonsen's image also involves a major assumption. The vessel in the picture can never contain less than nothing, so this assumes that positive experiences always equal or exceed negative ones. We could draw another version of the picture that didn't make this assumption, but we can also ask whether the assumption is reasonable: whether it is always or usually true that the sum of an animal's life is positive rather than

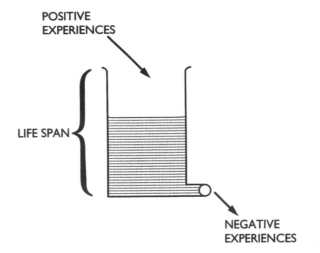

Fig. 4.3 Henrik Simonsen's depiction of the idea that the quality of life of an animal can be expressed as the sum of positive and negative experiences during its entire lifetime.[10] The model does not stand close analysis – for example, it cannot be used to compare animals with different lifespans – but the main idea is useful.

negative. This is similar to our main question, is an animal's life worth living?

There are some animals for which the assumption in Simonsen's picture seems to be wrong. Here is an extreme case. In 1988, researchers in the USA were using genetic engineering to investigate how mouse embryos grow.[11] They produced a type of mutant mouse that they dubbed Legless. Embryos of this type had legs that were almost completely undeveloped or severely abnormal, and their heads were also deformed. They died either before birth or shortly after. It would be difficult to conclude that the short lives of Legless mice were positive in terms of welfare.

It is possible that the lives of some longer-lived animals are also negative in this sense. Perhaps some farm animals, kept throughout their lives in atrocious conditions in countries where there is little or no legislation against cruelty, have lives that are not worth living. However, this is probably rare in countries that do have such legislation. Even another relatively extreme case, the rearing of broiler chickens and turkeys, does not yield such a conclusion. John Webster suggests that:

> Approximately one quarter of the heavy strains of broiler chicken and turkey are in chronic pain for approximately one third of their lives.[6]

Yet this means that three-quarters are not in pain (although they may have other welfare problems), and that the rest are free of pain for two thirds of their lives.

This is beginning to sound unpleasantly cold-blooded in its weighing and measuring of lives. It is beginning to sound complacent about the suffering of broilers, turkeys and other animals. It is not complacent. The message of this chapter is that we should concentrate on reducing such suffering, rather than necessarily reducing the number of animals with which we interact.

Overall, it is reasonable to conclude that most animals have lives that are worth living, that are better than never having been born, that are positive rather than negative. By analogy, if severely handicapped people are asked if they wish they'd never been born, most of them say no, they don't regret having lived. This conclusion about the lives of animals has wide implications, which we shall consider in the next section.

A future for cows

With many of the animals we keep – farm and laboratory animals, pets, zoo and circus animals – we could potentially reduce numbers, possibly even to zero.

Addressing this issue world-wide would be complicated. So let us consider a single country, and a single category of animals: farm animals. The rhetoric of 'Stop using animals', taken to its logical conclusion, would mean that such a country would have to phase out cattle and pigs, sheep and goats, chickens and turkeys. Perhaps in theory we could let them continue breeding, and treat them as pets, or wild animals, or something in between. But in practice we would have to reduce the numbers of these animals to only a handful.

We shall leave aside the question of whether this is practical (is it sustainable to make shoes from oil-based materials?) and the fact that it wouldn't free us from ethical concerns (rearing crops to eat also involves killing animals, because pests have to be controlled). We shall just consider the following question.

Would a country without cows be a better place from our point of view, from the cows' point of view, from the point of view of an impartial observer like the Martian invoked in Chapter 3? The answer is probably no, from all three points of view.

The most difficult of these viewpoints to address is that of the cows, because to ask a question from the 'point of view' of cows that are not yet born and that might never be born is dubious. There is an extensive discussion in philosophy about whether this sort of approach is valid: for example, whether we can have duties to future generations.[12] However, it does seem reasonable to say that if the majority of cows have lives that are worth living, that are positive rather than negative, then it is better *for the cows themselves* to be present than to be absent.

There is also room for argument about whether humans or impartial observers should prefer to phase out cows. One relevant point is that the methane produced by cows is a major contributor to global warming.[4] But this is more a matter of whether we should reduce the number of cows than of whether we should stop using them.

On the matter of using cows, even compromises would be difficult. It might seem that we could keep dairy cows for milk and not use them in any other way. But for cows to go on producing milk, they must go on producing calves – usually one calf each year. If we are not to be over-run with cattle, they have to be killed. If they have to be killed, why shouldn't we eat them?

When pushed in this way, most people would probably agree that our co-operative relationship should continue with some categories of animals – with farm animals and pets, for example. They may be uneasy about killing farm animals or completely opposed to killing, and we shall consider this below, but apart from this very important aspect of the relationship they would agree that there is a future for cows and for dogs and cats in our society. There would also be a majority in favour of zoos continuing, given the increasing emphasis on their role in conservation and education.

On the other hand, there are other categories of animal for which the same logic seems to be less persuasive, such as circus animals and, particularly, laboratory animals. The logic is indeed the same: even if the procedures carried out on laboratory animals are questionable, those procedures usually occupy only a small part of their lives. So it is not clear that phasing out laboratory animals would benefit laboratory animals. Yet most people probably feel that, if possible, there should be no such animals. Again, we shall leave aside the practical arguments implied by the phrase 'if possible' (except that they are considered briefly in Box 4.1).

Box 4.1   The three Rs

As long ago as 1959, William Russell and Rex Burch wrote a pamphlet for the Universities Federation for Animal Welfare[13] called *The Principles of Humane Experimental Technique*. They classified humane techniques in the following way. The three Rs are widely quoted, not only for laboratory animals but also for other categories.

Replacement	means the substitution for conscious living higher animals of insentient material
Reduction	means reduction in the numbers of animals used to obtain information of given amount and precision
Refinement	means any decrease in the incidence or severity of inhumane procedures applied to those animals which still have to be used

This contrast in attitude – that people see a future for cows, but not for laboratory mice – is at least partly a case of special pleading. We like cows, and we like having them around, more than we like mice. So we argue for their continued existence, not for their own sake but for ours: in other words, our 'uses' of cows are not limited to the meat and milk we get from them. We get much less pleasure, by contrast, from the thought of millions of mice in laboratories.

Secondly, however, the different attitude to cows and to laboratory mice may partly depend on common perceptions of the extent to which our relationship with different categories of animals can readily be seen as two-sided. We can imagine farmers treating farm animals with respect and providing for their needs (as far as possible) throughout their lives (Fig. 4.4). We find it difficult to imagine laboratory scientists behaving in the same way with their laboratory animals. Later chapters will consider whether this is fair. In brief, quite a lot of progress has been made in quite a lot of countries, with moves towards group housing for some laboratory animals and considerably more attention being paid to their welfare by institutions and by individual scientists and technicians – although there is still considerable room for progress. A similar story can be told for zoo and circus animals, as well as for farm animals and pets.

In any event, all these arguments support our main conclusion: that we should give more attention to the welfare of the animals in our care. The eighteenth century German philosopher Immanuel Kant emphasized that we should never use other people purely for our own ends – we should also pay regard to their ends, to their needs and desires.[14] Tom Regan extended this idea to animals, in establishing the principle of animal rights: he said that individuals 'must never be treated *merely as a means* to securing the best aggregate consequences'.[9] That is what we are saying here: that where we do use animals in a predominantly one-sided way we should stop doing so. There may be some cases where we can only achieve this by phasing out their use, reducing their numbers in a humane way, possibly to zero. In most cases, however, we can achieve the same aim by making the relationship more two-sided, more fair to the animals who are passive partners in the contract, rather than by getting rid of them. Of the three Rs listed in Box 4.1, we should give most emphasis to refinement of animal treatment (in laboratories and elsewhere) and less to replacement and reduction. There is a future for cows.

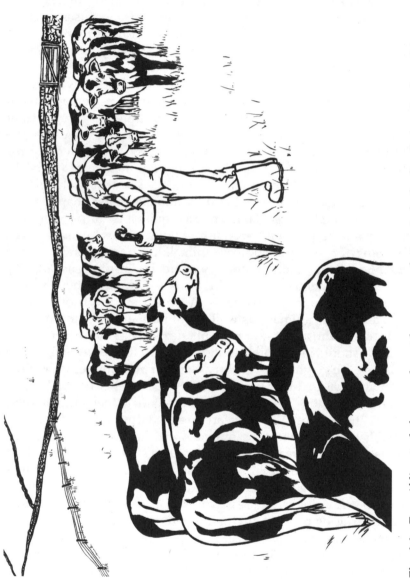

Fig. 4.4 Even if livestock farmers do not have as much time to look after their animals as this traditional sort of image would suggest, most are in the business because they like animals.

The tiger and the deer

It is not just the future of animals we keep that is problematic, it is that of all the animals in the world, because we are changing the environment even in the remotest places. Furthermore, humans benefit from many species of animal that we don't keep directly under our control, whether by hunting them for sport, killing them for food or appreciating them, as John Webster puts it, 'for their fearful symmetry and as symbols of freedom itself'.[6]

The title of this section is adapted from that of George Schaller's book *The Deer and the Tiger*,[15] because there are two main categories of wildlife in this context. First, there are species like the tiger that are approaching extinction either because people have killed so many or because of other human activities such as restriction of their habitat. As mentioned in Chapter 3, this may not be a question of animal welfare as such. Peter Sandøe and his colleagues point out that there is a widely held view:

> ... that the extinction of a species is something to be deplored not only because of its consequences for the welfare of humans or animals but as something that is *in itself* bad. If the blue whale becomes extinct this will not be a problem for animal welfare – the whales do not suffer from being extinct. Many humans will regret the loss, but it seems to reverse the true order of things to say that loss of a species is bad because it is regretted by humans. It seems that we should regret the loss of a species because its existence is in itself morally valuable. This seems to imply that we have duties to species and not (only) to individual animals.[16]

Indeed, duties to species and to individuals may be contradictory. Tom Regan has suggested that:

> If we had to choose between saving the last two members of an endangered species, or saving another individual who belonged to a species that was plentiful but whose death would be a greater *prima facie* harm to that individual than the harm that death would be to the two, then the rights view requires that we save the individual.[9]

But it's a fair bet that most people (and maybe even Regan among them) would plump for the last two tigers if it actually came down to it, rather than sticking rigidly to 'the rights view' (Fig. 4.5). This is one of the situations where people do not confine themselves to one restrictive ethical approach but find specific answers to specific problems – as outlined in Chapter 1. Given

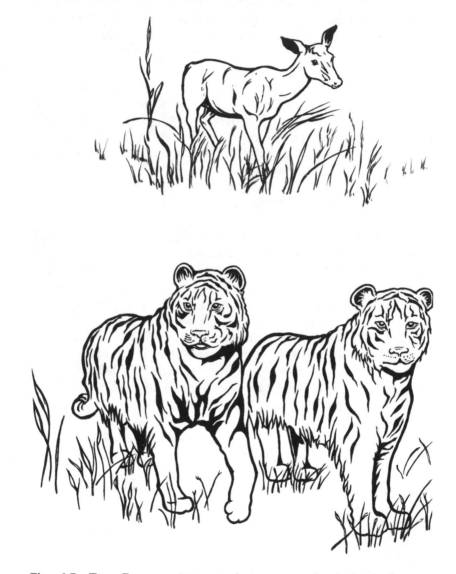

Fig. 4.5 Tom Regan points out that concern for individuals may sometimes favour common species such as deer rather than rare ones such as tigers. However, other views of our responsibilities include the need for conservation.

elements of concern for the tigers themselves (either their welfare or their rights), concern for the environment and concern for ourselves, people think that we should do more to prevent the extinction both of particular species, such as tigers, and of animal species in general.[17]

Secondly, there are species that tend to increase in numbers, like deer in many countries. Take red deer in the UK as an example. We have removed the natural predators of deer such as wolves and bears. So we have a choice. Either we manage the population: in other words, kill some deer each year to leave the remainder with a decent food supply. Or we leave them alone, in which case the population increases until more and more die of malnutrition in the winter. Society has chosen the former option, partly because the latter is just another, slower way of killing them and partly perhaps because there are other factors involved, such as the meat that can be obtained from shot animals.

Yet there are dilemmas. Choosing the best population size is a complex process: is it better to have fewer well-fed deer or a larger number of poorly fed individuals? Is it better from our point of view or from theirs? Deciding how excess deer are to be killed is also complex. A recent scientific report by Professor Patrick Bateson[18] showed that hunting with dogs causes suffering in deer. As a result, the UK's National Trust banned such hunting on its extensive land-holdings in the southwest of England. Unfortunately, farmers in some areas such as the Quantock Hills who supported hunting are now shooting deer, and it is likely that deer in the Quantocks will soon be wiped out.[19] Indeed, some animals move from this category – tending to increase in numbers – to the other category – in danger of extinction – because of just such exploitation on a larger scale. Whales are a notorious example, with many species threatened by over-exploitation.

Furthermore, some people still have qualms about the killing. A resident of Nottingham wrote to me recently to complain about the shooting of deer in a nearby park, by employees of the local council. Some children who visited the park regularly had even given some of them names, she said, and asked: 'Couldn't the deer be sterilized?' I pointed out that the deer would have to be tranquillized, and sterilization would be a chancy procedure. Management of a free-ranging herd, some of which were sterile, would be difficult, and there would still be the question of what to do with old animals. I also said that if deer had to be removed then shooting was the most humane way to do it: quick and painless. Perhaps the biggest mistake of the council had been in not explaining fully enough what it was doing and why. This takes us on to a major crunch issue: the killing itself.

Death is part of life

As we have seen – particularly in Chapter 1 – there are diverse opinions on killing. Let us concentrate on humane killing of animals under our control, for example farm and laboratory animals or deer in a park. Some philosophers believe that this is acceptable, while some believe that it is rarely so, and members of the public also disagree on this matter. Some of the factors that affect these opinions are considered in Box 4.2.

There is a major factor in this disagreement that has been widely overlooked. It is this: killing is too often considered in isolation, too often analysed separately from the rest of the animal's life. In our distress for the death of a human being we are regularly counselled to remember that death is part of life. Yet we frequently discuss the death of an animal without any reference to the life that went before. This argument does not mean for a moment that death is unimportant, just that it has to be seen in context.

For example, John Webster suggests in his book *Animal Welfare* that soul-searching over the killing of animals is mistaken:

> If we object, on grounds of conscience, to the killing of animals (or nominated species of animals) by man, we do not ensure the preservation of individual lives, we merely change the method of death. Pursuing this logic even more ruthlessly, if we elect not to eat animals, they will still get eaten.[6]

No. Webster's argument is more-or-less correct for wild animals, such as wild red deer, because even individuals that die of old age will be eaten. However, it is incorrect for farm animals. If we elect not to eat cows, the cows that are alive today will still get eaten, but fewer cows will be born in future. If we want to avoid responsibility for the deaths of animals under our control, we can do so by preventing them living at all. But as we have said, if the majority of these animals have lives that are worth living, that are positive rather than negative, preventing them living seems to be

Box 4.2   Is killing acceptable?

People disagree on whether it is acceptable to kill animals, and on which of the following characteristics are relevant to the decision:

Self-consciousness	It is commonly agreed that self-conscious animals can understand the concept of death and that it is generally wrong to kill them. DeGrazia, for example, concludes that 'The presumption against killing humans, great apes and dolphins is virtually absolute'.[20] For some philosophers, such as Singer, this is the only important characteristic.[21]
Sociality	Killing one individual may also affect other members of the group. Complexity and emotional depth of relationships vary between species, so it is likely that sociality is particularly important in self-conscious species. A detailed study of vervet monkeys, for example, suggested that they can feel fear and grief but not compassion or empathy,[22] whereas great apes may also be able to feel the latter emotions.
Sentience	Some argue that all animals capable of enjoyment have an interest in continuing to live and are therefore harmed by being killed. Tom Regan, for example, refers to sentient animals as 'experiencing subjects of a life'.[9]
Life	Respect for animals does not necessarily depend on their brain power and many people avoid killing any animals unnecessarily, however simple. Albert Schweitzer talked of 'extending the circle of our compassion to all living things'.[23]

a disadvantage for the animals themselves. Webster may be right that humane killing of animals under our control is ethically acceptable, but not for the reason he gives.

I personally believe that it is indeed ethically acceptable to give an animal life and then to end that life in a humane way. There is a long evolutionary and historical background to the co-operation between us and animals, and I do not believe it is appropriate to 'phase out' most of the animals that depend on us for life.

This approach may even be compatible with animal rights, if we give sufficient attention to the needs of the animals in giving them a reasonable life and if their rights are considered over their whole lifetimes, not just at the moment of death. The principal transgression of animal rights is not the killing itself, nor the using of animals, but the using of them *merely as a means* to our ends.

Some categories of animals under our control are declining in numbers, notably laboratory animals (Chapter 7). But for now there are laboratory animals, domestic animals and some other animals in our care. What are we going to do about it?

A good life and a gentle death

To improve animal welfare we must concentrate on how we affect animals, not on whether we do so – on providing good conditions while they are alive and careful euthanasia or careful slaughter when the time comes.

Careful slaughter is not a contradiction in terms. There is a slaughterhouse in Spain that uses a surprisingly low-key system.[24] They back a lorry load of pigs up to the door, let down the ramp, arrange hurdles to guide the animals into the building and let the pigs emerge from the lorry in their own time. Pigs are inquisitive animals, and sooner or later each one finds its way round the corner. There a slaughterman stands waiting with the electric tongs, stuns each pig as it arrives without restraining it and without fuss, fixes a hoist to its leg and sends it on its way. The system seems somehow sneaky but it is certainly humane. As it happens this is a small business – the owner is involved in every aspect of the work – with a particular interest in meat quality, but similar care can and should be applied in large-scale facilities. Considerable improvements have been made in the design of facilities for the handling and slaughter of farm animals, particularly by the American behavioural scientist

Temple Grandin. She points out that meat quality, labour efficiency and animal welfare are correlated:

> Gentle handling in well-designed facilities will minimize stress levels, improve efficiency and maintain good meat quality. Rough handling or poorly designed equipment is detrimental to both animal welfare and meat quality. Progressive slaughter plant managers recognize the importance of good handling practices. Constant management supervision is required to maintain high humane standards.[25]

On the other hand, Peter Singer goes further in arguing that animals should be allowed a decent life. He does not condemn slaughter as such but nevertheless advocates vegetarianism.

> It is not practically possible to rear animals for food on a large scale without inflicting considerable suffering ... So we must ask ourselves, not: Is it ever right to eat meat? but: Is it right to eat this meat? Here I think that those who are opposed to the needless killing of animals and those who oppose only the infliction of suffering must join together and give the same, negative answer ... Vegetarianism is a form of boycott ... Until we boycott meat, and all other products of animal factories, we are, each one of us, contributing to the continued existence, prosperity and growth of factory farming and all the other cruel practices used in rearing animals for food.[21]

Some people agree with Singer (or with Regan on animal rights) and feel a duty to become vegetarian. This may be important for their personal integrity and it may also help to publicize the problems of intensive farming (see Chapter 8). Unfortunately it does not improve animal welfare. It reduces the numbers of animals being reared for meat, but it does not improve the conditions of those that continue to be reared and slaughtered.

Consider Singer's statement again: 'It is not practically possible to rear animals for food on a large scale without inflicting considerable suffering.' As it stands, this is a counsel of despair, because animals will continue to be reared for food on a large scale for the foreseeable future. But the statement is arguable: its strength depends on what is meant by 'considerable'. The contention of the present book is that we must reduce the suffering of animals reared for food, and of other animals as well. We must ensure that animals in our care do not undergo 'considerable suffering'. We must strive to give them a good life and a gentle death.

Conclusions

- Our relationship with animals is two-sided and we have a responsibility to look after their interests as well as our own. Legislation and language about owning animals are not the primary factors in determining our behaviour to animals but do affect attitudes.
- Most animals have lives that are worth living and we should concentrate on improving their lives rather than on reducing their numbers. This applies most obviously to farm animals and pets, but also to zoo, circus and laboratory animals.
- Our influence on the environment means that we also have responsibility for wild animals, including conservation of rare species and management of common ones – which may involve culling.
- Killing should not be considered in isolation but in the context of the animal's whole life. For us to take responsibility for killing, and to carry out that killing as humanely as possible, is compatible with giving animals decent lives up to that point. An exception where killing is almost never acceptable is great apes, because of their highly developed consciousness and sociality.

References

1. Budiansky, S. (1992) *The Covenant of the Wild: Why Animals Chose Domestication*. Weidenfeld & Nicolson, London.
2. Coppinger, R.P. & Smith, C.K. (1983) The domestication of evolution. *Environmental Conservation*, **10**, 283–92.
3. Morey, D.F. (1994) The early evolution of the domestic dog. *American Scientist*, **82**, 336–47.
4. Rifkin, J. (1992) *Beyond Beef: The Rise and Fall of the Cattle Culture*. Dutton, New York.
5. Photograph courtesy of Edinburgh Zoo.
6. Webster, A.J.F. (1994) *Animal Welfare: A Cool Eye Towards Eden*. Blackwell, Oxford.
7. Hearne, V. (1982) *Adam's Task: Calling Animals by Name*. Vintage, New York.

8. Brooman, S. & Legge, D. (1997) *Law Relating to Animals*. Cavendish, London.
9. Regan, T. (1983) *The Case for Animal Rights*. University of California Press, Berkeley.
10. Simonsen, H.B. (1996) Assessment of animal welfare by a holistic approach: behaviour, health and measured opinion. *Acta Agriculturae Scandinavica, Section A, Animal Science, Supplementum*, **27**, 91–6.
11. McNeish, J.D., Scott, W.J.Jr & Potter, S.S. (1988) Legless, a novel mutation found in PHT1-1 transgenic mice. *Science*, **241**, 837–9.
12. Parfit, D. (1982) Future generations: further problems. *Philosophy and Public Affairs*, **11**, 2.
13. Russell, W.M.S. & Burch, R. (1959 reissued 1992) *The Principles of Humane Experimental Technique*. Universities Federation for Animal Welfare, Potters Bar, UK.
14. Kant, I. (1786) *Grundlegung zur Metaphysik der Sitten*. Hartnoch, Riga.
15. Schaller, G.B. (1967) *The Deer and the Tiger: A Study of Wildlife in India*. University of Chicago Press, Chicago.
16. Sandøe, P., Crisp, R. & Holtug, N. (1997) Ethics. In *Animal Welfare* (eds M.C. Appleby & B.O. Hughes), pp. 3–17. CAB International, Wallingford, UK.
17. Rolston, H. (1989) The value of species. In *Animal Rights and Human Obligations* (eds T. Regan & P. Singer), pp. 252–5. Prentice Hall, Englewood Cliffs, NJ.
18. Bateson, P.P.G. (1997) *The Behavioural and Physiological Effects of Culling Red Deer*. Report to the Council of the National Trust.
19. Anonymous (1997) Article in *The Independent* newspaper, 25th November.
20. DeGrazia, D. (1996) *Taking Animals Seriously: Mental Life and Moral Status*. Cambridge University Press, Cambridge.
21. Singer, P. (1975) *Animal Liberation*. New York Review of Books, New York.
22. Cheney, D.L. & Seyfarth, R.M. (1990) *How Monkeys See the World: Inside the Mind of Another Species*. University of Chicago Press, Chicago.
23. Schweitzer, A. (1933) *My Life and Thought: An Autobiography* (trans. C.T. Campion). Allen & Unwin, London.
24. Professor Colin Whittemore, Institute of Ecology and Resource Management, University of Edinburgh, personal communication.
25. Grandin, T. (1993) Handling and welfare of livestock in slaughter plants. In *Livestock Handling and Transport* (ed. T. Grandin), pp. 289–311. CAB International, Wallingford, UK.

Chapter 5
Made in our image: Selection and modification of animals

The chosen few

Given that we keep animals, how do we change them? Are all domestic animals monsters of our own creation, or are some of the Frankenstein stories exaggerated?

Firstly we must consider the base material. It is remarkable that the vast numbers of domestic animals world-wide come from only a handful of species: around 20 mammals, 10 birds and a few others such as the carp, the honey bee and the silk moth. Even the species we exploit in other ways like hunting are relatively few in number. Some societies do use more – for example, the Chinese eat more varieties of animal than most – but even they rely on the same few species for the bulk of their use.

In the millennia before domestication began, people lived by hunting and gathering and concentrated on species that were most abundant or easiest to catch. A survey of Palaeolithic and Mesolithic sites across Europe found that 91% had remains of red deer, 83% of pigs and 61% of both cattle and roe deer.[1] Of these, people domesticated pigs and cattle but not deer. Deer have two disadvantages. Firstly they have antlers, which are even more dangerous than the horns of cattle and the teeth of pigs. Secondly, they are difficult to tame. Roe deer in particular are solitary or live in pairs in the wild; they cannot be kept in groups. Red deer are farmed today but this involves sawing the antlers off and using high fences to stop them escaping.

So there were two main criteria for domestication: usefulness and feasibility. The species that were domesticated had characteristics that made domestication possible, especially behaviour. They lived in groups. Once tame, they accepted humans as bosses of those groups. They were adaptable to varied

87

environments. Because these characteristics were necessary, they were mostly related. Fifteen of the domestic mammals are in the group called ungulates – the horse, cow, sheep, pig, camel and so on. Exceptions are the dog and cat, the rabbit, rat and mouse. All but one of the domestic birds are in two groups: the pheasants (including the chicken, turkey and quail) and the waterfowl (duck and goose). The odd one out is the pigeon (Fig. 5.1).

Domestication is not just tameness: it involves genetic change from the wild ancestors. This is inevitable, partly because the animals live in a new environment and the characteristics needed to survive and prosper are different, and partly because change is bound to accumulate in small populations. Even zoo animals diverge from their wild relatives over a number of generations. Some of the most striking changes in domestic species are by-products of captivity, for example changes in colour. Wild animals are generally camouflaged, and odd-coloured individuals don't survive very long, but those born in captivity may not only survive but pass their colour on to subsequent generations.

However, the genetic change was not all a matter of chance. There was one other important feature of the animals that became our domestic stock: most of them mated promiscuously rather than pairing for life. This meant that people could choose which individuals to pair with each other – or put them together at random – and still get offspring.

From the earliest times people must have kept and mated animals that were more useful, or more convenient, or more pleasing than others. If you had two bull calves, you'd kill the aggressive one to eat and keep the docile one, which would in due course become a father. Offspring resembled their parents both physically and in behaviour, and change accumulated over the generations. Some of this process was unintentional: you killed the aggressive bull because it was a nuisance, not because you thought about whether its offspring would be aggressive. But some of the process was certainly intentional, because people must always have been aware of similarities between parents and offspring. There is a clear account in the Bible, from about 3500 years ago, of just such awareness. Jacob was in charge of Laban's sheep and wanted the strongest lambs for himself:

Jacob said to Laban 'Let me take every speckled or spotted sheep, every dark-coloured lamb and every spotted or speck-led goat. They will be my wages.' Then Jacob took fresh-cut

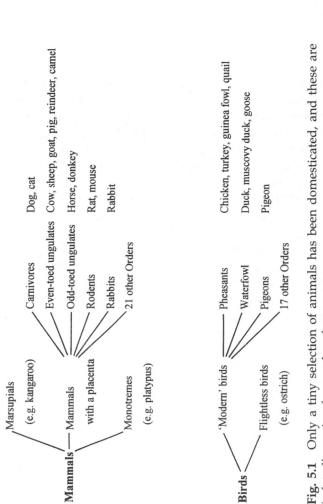

Fig. 5.1 Only a tiny selection of animals has been domesticated, and these are 'related', coming from only a few groups.

branches and made white stripes on them by peeling the bark. When the flocks were in heat and came to drink, they mated in front of the branches and they bore young that were streaked or speckled or spotted. Whenever the stronger females were in heat, Jacob would place the branches in front of the animals so that they would mate near the branches, but if the animals were weak, he would not place them there. So the weak animals went to Laban and the strong ones to Jacob.[2]

The account also reminds us that understanding of the processes involved was incomplete: the fact that spotted lambs were born was certainly independent of whether their mothers saw spotted branches. Understanding of genetics only dawned at the beginning of the twentieth century. Nevertheless, huge changes were achieved in some species. Pigs were bred so fat that their bellies scraped the ground. Pigeons and dogs were diversified on a whim: it is difficult to believe that pouters and fantails (Fig. 5.2) or pugs and pointers are members of the same species. The effects on welfare of such changes will be discussed below.

Yet other species changed remarkably little – sheep, goats and camels are not so different from wild animals – and even the most bizarre creations have more in common with their ancestors than might be apparent. This is for the very reason that they were domesticated in the first place – they had useful characteristics. This applies particularly to behaviour. If they are given the chance, domestic animals behave very like their wild relatives.

Until recently, many people assumed that domestic animals were degenerate. For example, there was a myth that they had small brains. However, this arose from a simple mistake: brain size was compared between, say, a fattening pig and a wild boar of the same *size*, forgetting that the domestic pig was younger. Juliet Clutton-Brock made this mistake, saying that 'In most domestic mammals the size of the brain becomes smaller relative to the size of the body'.[4] On the contrary, the size of the body becomes larger relative to the size of the brain. At the same *age*, the pig and the boar have brains of about the same size (Fig. 5.3).

Similarly, it was common to suggest that animals kept in intensive housing must get used to it over the generations. According to this argument, keeping pigs in stalls wasn't cruel: it was assumed that commercial pigs no longer had the same needs and desires as wild boars. This argument was thoroughly

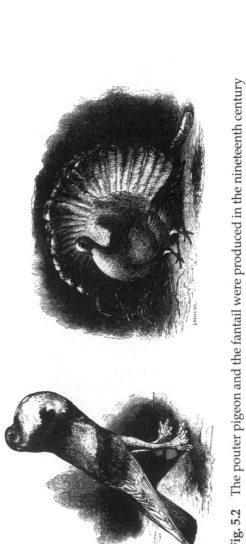

Fig. 5.2   The pouter pigeon and the fantail were produced in the nineteenth century by artificial selection from a common ancestor. Such changes contributed to the evidence accumulated by Darwin in developing his theory of evolution; these illustrations are from one of his books.[3]

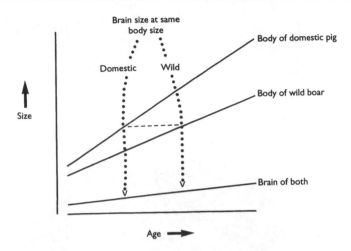

Fig. 5.3 At the same body size, a domestic pig has a smaller brain than a wild boar. But it is more appropriate to compare them at the same age, and then their brains are the same size.

scotched by Alex Stolba and my late colleague Professor David Wood-Gush. They took normal commercial pigs and released them in a large hillside enclosure outside Edinburgh called the Pig Park:

> Despite the fact that adults in the Pig Park had been reared under intensive conditions, they showed that domestication and rearing conditions had not affected their potential to show a rich repertoire of behaviour. Indeed, the behaviour ... resembled that of the European wild boar in wild or semi-wild conditions.[5]

Pigs spent much of the day foraging for food. They moved around in family groups (Fig. 5.4). When sows were ready to give birth they went off on their own and built a nest. In short, modern pigs had all the instincts of wild animals.

With hindsight it was obvious. There are thousands of feral pigs in the Australian outback and in the southern USA.[6] Domestic pigs can survive in the wild – as can other species such as dogs and cats – and to do that they need all their instincts. Many of those instincts are thwarted in commercial conditions, as we shall see in the next chapters.

So our domestic animals are a mixed bag. We have changed

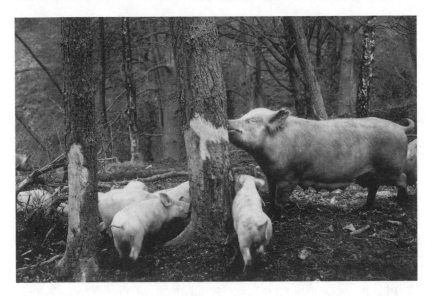

Fig. 5.4 Modern pigs have retained all the instrincts of their ancestor, the wild boar. This sow in the Edinburgh Pig Park is eating bark, and her piglets are learning to forage. Photograph courtesy of Ruth Newberry.

some of their features considerably, which causes problems, but we have left others mostly unchanged and that causes problems too. We may be able to solve these problems, but first we need to be aware of them. For illustration, let us consider one farm animal in more detail: the chicken. Remember that 'chicken' is used here to mean a domestic fowl of either sex and any age.

A history of hens

Chickens are the descendants of Red Jungle Fowl, which still strut and scrape in the forests of South and South-East Asia.[7] They were domesticated well over 8000 years ago, but many of them have changed very little: old-fashioned farmyard birds look just like Jungle Fowl. They will interbreed given the chance, and biologists classify chickens as a subspecies rather than a separate species.

One reason for this relative stability is that chickens haven't been kept for one purpose throughout their history, so they haven't been selected on consistent criteria. People have always eaten them and their eggs now and again, but for centuries the cocks were more important than the hens: they were kept for cockfighting or for crowing or for colourful plumage.[8] Cock-fighting was still common in eighteenth century Europe, and is still practised in some other parts of the world. Many farms then had a few chickens but they were still small and the hens laid only a couple of clutches of ten or a dozen eggs each year. Two developments followed. Firstly, breeding for larger size and for higher egg production started. Secondly, distinct breeds were produced. For example, by 1810 there was a breed in England called The Large.

In the nineteenth century there was a boom in poultry shows and societies, and poultry farming left the farmyard to become an industry. By the middle of the twentieth century the best-known breeds were established, such as Leghorns, selected for egg production, and Rhode Island Reds, kept for both meat and eggs.[9] For the rest of this section we shall concentrate on hens kept for egg production – often called layers. Meat birds – broilers – will be considered in the next section.

Fifty years ago welfare problems for layers were common, but most were surmounted by technical advances. For example, hens were now laying eggs on two days out of every three, which required a lot of calcium for the egg shells. Much of this came from the bones, and birds often became unable to stand – a condition euphemistically called layer fatigue. The problem was reduced, though, by improved methods of feeding. It was also limited by another feature of poultry biology that hadn't chan-ged. In contrast to domestic pigs and cattle, which breed at any time of year, chickens are still strongly affected by the seasons.[7] Jungle Fowl only lay eggs in spring and summer, so the chicks hatch when there's plenty of food, and until 1950 or so hens still got a respite by producing fewer eggs during the short days of autumn and winter.

Since then hens have come under increased pressure. Some of this is from artificial genetic selection, using ever more sophis-ticated techniques. Some of it, however, is from other technical approaches, applied precisely because selection has not been successful. It has not been possible to breed hens insensitive to daylength, so they are now kept in houses with controlled day-length, to persuade them that it is forever spring. It has not been possible to produce breeds that lay every day, so breeds such as Leghorns and Rhode Island Reds are rarely used now. Instead producers cross different breeds, which produces the effect called hybrid vigour. What do you get if you cross a Leghorn with a Rhode Island? More eggs.

Hens today walk a welfare tightrope. They lay over 300 eggs in a year, which needs a very delicate balance of the body's systems. If all goes well the balance is maintained, but it can easily be disturbed. A large proportion of hens have cancer of the oviduct, caused by the high concentrations of sex hormones that are now permanent instead of temporary.[10] Many have weak bones, that break easily when the birds are handled at the end of their lives.[11]

But as we've established, not all these problems are genetic. The point is this: breeding has produced some problems, but it could nevertheless reduce others. It should be possible to breed hens less responsive to daylength, and give them more freedom. It should be possible to breed birds less susceptible to cancer and broken bones. If we could go back to using pure breeds, instead of creating birds anew in every generation, they could be adapted to their housing.

This sounds an over-technological approach to a technological difficulty – setting a thief to catch a thief. Couldn't we just go back to old-fashioned, less intensive production? That question will be discussed in the next two chapters but the answer, simply, is no, not without huge changes – such as no-one eating eggs at all unless they or their neighbours keep hens.

Anyway, genetic selection is not intrinsically evil: it can be regarded as just a tool that can be used well or ill. Many of the changes made to domestic animals have been solely for human benefit, and animal welfare has suffered. Yet if breeding was carried out for the animals' sake as well as for humans a reasonable compromise could be reached. We shall examine this possibility – and the welfare problems that make it necessary – in the other main category of chickens, the birds reared for meat.

The slippery slope

Until after the Second World War there were no breeds of chickens kept just for meat production. Birds reared for meat grew slowly unless they were fattened by force-feeding. This practice is now illegal in many countries, although used on ducks and geese in France and Belgium to produce fatty livers (foie gras) for paté. Then in the 1950s specialist meat birds were developed that became known as broiler chickens.[9] This was achieved using methods similar to those for egg production:

selection for fast growth, crossing of breeds to get hybrid vigour and development of new feeding methods.

In practical terms the success of these techniques has been spectacular. In the post-war period a meat bird took over 13 weeks to grow to 2 kg and cost about £40 in today's money. Today it takes less than 6 weeks (Fig. 5.5) and costs less than £2.

But we must realize that farmers do not generally make greater profits as a result. Certainly the main motive has been economic, but that must be seen in the context of competition between producers. Each strives to cut costs and to market their product as cheaply as possible, to stay in the race. The main economic benefit has been to consumers, who now buy chicken more cheaply. Whether consumers really want their chicken to be produced more cheaply is a question for Chapter 8.

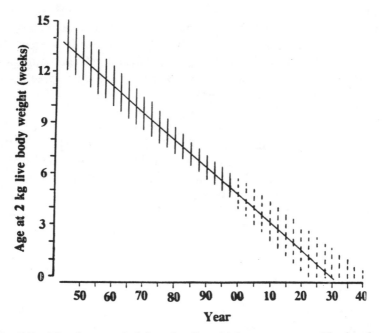

Fig. 5.5 The time needed for a broiler chicken to grow to 2 kg has been reduced steadily over the last 50 years, as shown by the sloping line on this graph (the vertical lines show maximum and minimum values). If similar reduction was possible in future, as shown by the part of the graph with dashed vertical lines, chicks would eventually be 2 kg just after hatching! But there must be limitations on this process that will soon prevent further reduction.[12]

In welfare terms there are two major problems associated with growth rate. First, many broilers have leg abnormalities: bone or joint diseases that prevent them walking normally. A survey in 1992 by scientists from the University of Bristol[13] concluded that 26% of commercial broilers were in chronic pain before slaughter – and some of the worst cases had already been culled by that time. John Webster says that:

> Most of these conditions can be attributed, in simple terms, to birds that have grown too heavy for their limbs and/or become so distorted in shape as to impose unnatural stresses on their joints.[14]

Secondly, the parents of these birds are kept permanently hungry. They cannot be fed freely because they would grow so obese that their health would decline and they couldn't mate properly. They are given between quarter and half of what they would eat given the chance and they are eager to eat at all times.[15]

These problems have arisen gradually, generation by generation over the last 50 years: a long and slippery slope. Nobody looked ahead 50 years ago and foresaw what a 1990s broiler would be like. Imagine for a moment that a 1990s bird had been introduced suddenly in the 1940s (Fig. 5.6), perhaps by genetic engineering. It wouldn't have been allowed: the problems would have seemed too great. But the problems have grown stage by stage, and there were no laws, no procedures that said 'Thus far and no farther.'

Such procedures are now being developed, at least in the UK. In parallel with the Bristol study, the Farm Animal Welfare Council (FAWC) reviewed broiler welfare and concluded that:

> The current level of leg problems in broilers is unacceptable. We recommend that steps should be taken to ensure that there is a significant reduction in the numbers and severity of leg problems. It will be the responsibility of the industry to achieve this objective and ... if no reduction in leg problems is found, we may recommend the introduction of legislation.[17]

The broiler industry has responded. It has changed the management of young birds, giving them shorter days, which reduces overeating during their initial, rapid growth. At the European Symposium on Poultry Welfare in The Netherlands in June 1997

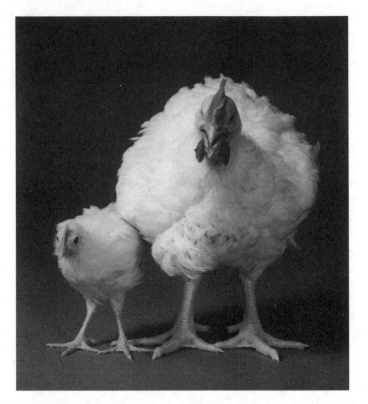

Fig. 5.6 These chickens are the same age, 6 weeks old. When the one on the left is mature it will lay eggs for sale. The broiler on the right is ready to be slaughtered for meat.[16]

speakers from the industry said that the incidence of leg problems has declined as a result, although no figures have been published to confirm this.

Furthermore, breeders have also started to select for leg strength. As we said, genetic selection can be used to benefit animals as well as humans, and it is known that many leg problems can be reduced by selection.[18] Why has this knowledge not been put into practice? Because selecting for leg strength slows down progress on growth rate. The balance sheet is negative: the economic benefit of stronger legs is less than the economic loss of slower growth (or not-so-much-faster growth). So breeders are still selecting for growth rate – and achieving it. Broilers are still reaching the desired slaughter weights younger and younger each year. It remains to be seen whether the balance breeders are attempting – to select for both leg strength and growth rate – is tipped sufficiently far in favour of the animals to eliminate most of the problems. FAWC will soon be reviewing their progress and it may still be that legislation should follow.

There has been less attention to the hunger of breeding birds. It may be that management can also help here. For example, just as tethers and stalls have been banned for hungry sows (as we saw in Chapter 2), giving broiler parents more space and varied conditions might reduce the stress of food restriction. An alternative idea was that it might be better to give birds large amounts of bulky food rather than small amounts of concentrates, but unfortunately this does not seem to reduce hunger.[19] Anyway, the problem also needs to be tackled directly – and this again involves genetics. What we need are birds that are fertile without food restriction. It may be possible to select for this directly.[20] One other approach that is being used in France, and deserves more attention elsewhere, is use of what are called dwarf birds.[18] Dwarfs look perfectly normal, and they remain fertile when fed as much as they want to eat, but they are smaller than usual. However, the condition is caused by a single gene and does not appear in the offspring – which therefore grow like any other broilers.

Again it is not clear whether producers can make changes like this in a competitive market, without risking going out of business. It may be that legislation is needed to give the competitors a 'level playing field', enforcing change for all of them. But it is clear that genetics can be used to increase animal welfare[21] as well as human profit. Broilers and their parents – and sows, and dairy cows, and other animals selected intensively for production over the generations – can and must be pushed back up the slippery slope.

The long jump

If traditional selective breeding sometimes takes us gradually down a slope, genetic engineering seems like a long jump into the unknown – or worse, into horrors that we can foresee. In fact, fewer Frankenstein monsters have been produced so far than the fear of the unknown might suggest. However, there are certainly some monsters in the story, and as new discoveries are announced almost daily, more may possibly be waiting round the corner. This is good reason to demand vigilant control over future developments, and possibly more legal restrictions.

Some of the worst monsters produced by genetic engineering were the Beltsville pigs. In the mid-1980s, scientists working at Beltsville Agricultural Station in the USA inserted extra genes for growth hormone into the DNA of pigs.[22] The extra hormone made the pigs grow faster, as intended, but it also disrupted the whole balance of the growth process so that they developed gross arthritis and other problems. The photographs of these pigs are disturbing (Fig. 5.7).

The lesson has been learned. People sometimes refer to the Beltsville pigs as if genetic engineers and farmers would like to put such monsters into large scale production, but of course that isn't true. On the contrary, the suffering of those few pigs – while horrible for them – acted as a warning and a brake on developments in this area of science. Expectations of improving growth rate in farm animals are now less than they were – as shown in Box 5.1.

Unfortunately, another area of work has also declined recently. It was hoped that genetic engineering could make animals more

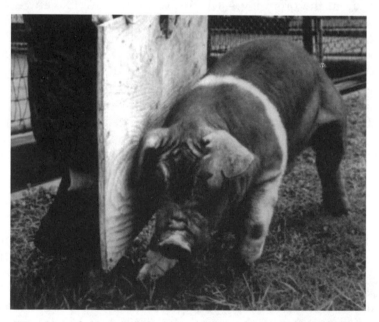

Fig. 5.7 One of the Beltsville pigs produced by genetic engineering, with extra genes for growth hormone. They grew rapidly but had many problems such as arthritis.[23]

Box 5.1   Genetic engineering of animals: main areas of research

The main welfare effects of the most common lines of work in each category are shown, although there will be exceptions in each case.[24] Welfare is interpreted here in terms of animal minds and bodies; implications of genetic engineering for animal natures are considered in the next section.

	Examples	Welfare	Status
Farm animals for agricultural products			
Growth rate	Beltsville pigs	**Negative**	Less active
Disease resistance		**Positive**	Less active
Special products	Herman the bull	Neutral	Developing
Farm animals for biomedical products			
Pharmaceuticals	Tracy the sheep	Neutral	Active
Organs	Pigs for hearts	Neutral	Developing
Experimental animals			
Understanding biology	Dolly the sheep	Neutral	Active
Understanding human disease	Oncomice	**Negative**	Active

---

resistant to disease – for the benefit of both the animals and their owners – but this has not yet been successful.

Most other areas of work on farm animals have surprisingly little effect on their welfare. Here are three examples. In the first, some workers are trying to modify milk, or other products from animals. In The Netherlands, a bull called Herman has been given the gene for a human protein.[25] This has no effect in him, but when he passes it on to his daughters they produce milk that is more digestible for babies. It is even possible that the welfare of the cows might be improved, as they may be less susceptible to udder infection (mastitis).

Secondly, sheep have been modified to produce medicines in their milk. The first world-famous sheep at the Roslin Institute near Edinburgh was called Tracy. She was altered by genetic engineering to have a chemical in her milk that can be used to treat emphysema in humans.[26] The medicine from Tracy's successors is now being tested in clinical trials.

Thirdly, pigs are being altered to allow their hearts and other organs to be used in transplants to humans.[27] This involves giving them a human gene so that the patient's immune system doesn't immediately reject the graft.

All of this work is controversial, and some of the ethical issues will be discussed in the next section. All of the animals concerned are treated differently from other farm animals – for example, they are often kept in isolation – but none of them are monsters. A cow or a sheep producing a slightly modified form of milk doesn't suffer as a direct result of that change, and neither does a pig with a human gene in its cells. The same is true for the most famous animal of them all – Dolly the sheep. Since Dolly was cloned at the Roslin Institute[28] the whole world has been discussing the issues involved, but it remains true that she could be shown to the press without embarrassment – a healthy, normal-looking sheep.

The same is not true, however, for all experimental animals. Legless mice were mentioned in Chapter 4 and there are many others as horrific as the Beltsville pigs. Mice are most commonly used, and the most notorious are the Harvard Oncomice.[29] These have been altered genetically to make them susceptible to cancer, and sure enough they develop various growths and other problems, often grossly obtrusive and debilitating. Not all mice used in genetic engineering suffer in this way, but a considerable number of deformed or sick animals are intentionally produced on a regular basis.

Why is this work done? Primarily because an understanding of how the body works and of what can go wrong may help in the prevention and treatment of disease in humans. Some scientists say that the understanding is important in itself – that an increase in knowledge is sufficient justification. However, in most countries permission is only given for work causing suffering if it also has potential benefits. Our society has generally taken the view that costs for animals can be offset by benefits for humans, and this sort of work isn't new. Before the Oncomice existed, mice were given cancer by other methods such as heavy doses of X-rays, and those mice suffered just as much. The work has to be seen in perspective. In the UK there were 547 000 mutant and transgenic mice produced in 1997.[30] That is a lot of mice, but it is only one for every 110 people, and the number is dwarfed by the 520 million broilers reared and killed each year.

But as with other arguments about 'perspective', this is absolutely no cause for complacency. A proportion of those half-million mice undergo suffering, and whatever number that represents is too many if their suffering can be avoided. Furthermore, the number of such mice produced is increasing each year. Consider again the idea that costs for animals can be offset by benefits for humans. We saw in Chapter 1 that many people feel this utilitarian approach has been weighted too heavily in favour of humans. Furthermore, many people combine elements of an animal rights view with their utilitarianism. They 'would say that there are certain things one may not do to animals, no matter how beneficial the consequences, for example causing the animals to experience intense suffering'.[31] This suggests that there should be increased stringency in the vetting of experiments, whether they are on genetic engineering or other approaches that cause animal suffering. The bodies that do such vetting (usually the Home Office in the UK) should give more weight to the suffering, compared to the potential human benefits. Indeed, perhaps they should consider other approaches to achieving similar benefits, such as preventative medicine. Perhaps they should increase the public debate on such criteria. We shall discuss this again in Chapter 9.

Calls for a blanket ban on genetic engineering are not justified purely on grounds of animal suffering. Many genetic modifications cause little or no suffering, and certainly less than many results of conventional genetic selection. Ironically, the 'instant' nature of genetic engineering also allows careful consideration of its consequences, in contrast to the slippery slope of generation-by-generation selection. However, there is still a lot of disturbing work going on, causing severe suffering to many animals. Such work needs much more debate, much more justification and – if such justification is not forthcoming – much more restriction.

It ain't natural

There is another aspect of the debate about genetic selection and genetic engineering that is only indirectly concerned with disease, deformity or suffering. So far we have concentrated on functions and feelings – on animal bodies and minds. What about animal natures? In Chapter 2 we noted that many people are concerned about unnatural environments for animals, and they have the same concern about genetic change: it's not natural.

Michael Fox makes this point in relation to genetic engineering, but it applies equally well to conventional genetic selection. In the following passage he borrows the Greek word *telos* from the writings of Aristotle, to mean more-or-less what we have been calling 'animal nature':

> The *telos* or 'beingness' of an animal is its intrinsic nature coupled with the environment in which it is able to develop and experience life. We can harm the *telos* in many ways, for example through environmental, genetic, surgical and phar-macological manipulation. To contend that we can enhance the natural *telos* of an animal – and thus by extension believe that we can improve upon nature – is *hubris*. Genetic engineering makes it possible to breach the genetic boundaries that nor-mally separate the genetic material of totally unrelated species. This means that the *telos*, or inherent nature, of animals can be so drastically modified (for example by inserting elephant growth hormone genes into cattle) as to radically change the entire direction of evolution, and primarily toward human ends at that. Is that aspect of the animal's *telos* we refer to as the genome and the gene pool of each species not to be respected and not worthy of moral consideration?[32]

Fox makes one technical error: inserting elephant growth hormone genes into cattle wouldn't be an appropriate way of making cattle grow more. It is the amount of growth hormone that is important, not the species it comes from, but his point is still clear.

Peter Sandøe and his colleagues describe this approach as a demand to respect the integrity of species, rather than just of individual animals. However, they point out problems with the approach:

> The first problem is the question of what is special about the genetic structures which exist right now. Throughout evolu-tion genetic structures have changed continuously. There is no stage in evolution at which animal species have reached their 'final' development. To say that the present genetic make-up is special is arbitrary – like saying that art and lit-

erature have reached their final points and should not change further.

The second problem with this view is that breeding for increased health – for hens resistant to Marek's disease or pigs without malignant hyperthermia – is usually considered a good thing. Although this may be seen as a remedy of damages in the genepool established during genetic selection of high yielding domestic species, such breeding may eradicate genotypes disposed to certain illnesses and secure the health of domestic stock. However, the demand to respect species-integrity will also tell against selective breeding: like transgenesis, selective breeding will result in significant genetic changes in species. This tells against the idea of species-integrity.[31]

The concept of naturalness is hard to pin down, in relation to environments, to genes and to the bodies they control. But as we said in Chapter 2, the point about respecting animal natures is not specific. It is a question of treating cows as cows, rather than as machines or humans or economic units. It is a corrective to the overemphasis on specific details suggested by people concerned only with animal minds and bodies.

There is no clear consensus here. Michael Reiss and Roger Straughan – a biologist and a philosopher writing on the ethics of genetic engineering – discuss work on turkeys[33] intended to increase their egg production by preventing them becoming broody (Fig. 5.8):

> At present, farmers try to 'shock' female turkeys out of broody behaviour by exposing them to bright lights or by making them stand on wires, so that they are unable to settle down and brood. It could be argued that genetically engineering turkeys so that the females do not show broody behaviour will be to the benefit of the animals' welfare. Of course, this line of reasoning is open to disputation on the grounds that two wrongs don't make a right ... [This work involves] an excessively instrumental view of living creatures ... All poultry should be able to engage in nest building and at least some brooding behaviour.[34]

By contrast Bernard Rollin, a powerful advocate for animal welfare, thinks that it is acceptable to change animal natures:

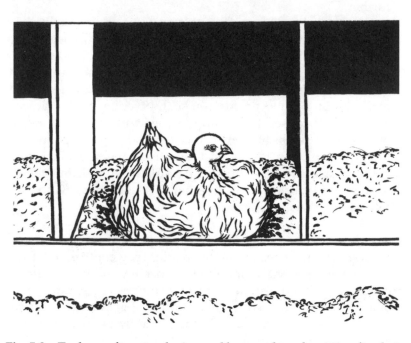

Fig. 5.8   Turkeys often stop laying and become broody, sitting firmly in a nest box as if incubating a clutch of eggs. This is a natural part of reproductive behaviour but is a problem for commercial production.

Consider a case where one might be tempted to change the telos of an animal – chickens kept in battery cages for efficient, high-yield egg production. It is now recognised that such a production system frustrates numerous significant aspects of chicken behavior under natural conditions, including nesting behavior, and that frustration of this basic need or drive results in a mode of suffering for the animals. Let us suppose that we have identified the gene or genes that code for the drive to nest. In addition, suppose we can ablate that gene or substitute a gene that creates a new kind of chicken, one that achieves satisfaction by laying an egg in a cage ... Have we done something morally wrong?

I would argue that we have not. A key feature of the new ethic for animals I have described is concern for preventing animal suffering and augmenting animal happiness, which I have argued involves satisfaction of telos ... If changing animals by genetic engineering is the only way to assure that they do not suffer, people will surely accept that strategy, though doubtless with some reluctance.[36]

This difference of views does not, in this case, mainly stem from different approaches to animal welfare: the authors seem to agree on the importance of animal natures. In fact their end-points are not as divergent as they initially appear. Reiss and Straughan conclude that the work on turkeys is ethically questionable, but point out that it may in practice improve welfare. Rollin suggests that the hypothetical work on hens would reduce suffering, but that the public would have reservations in accepting it. Most importantly, they agree that animal welfare must be explicitly taken into account in the assessment of whether genetic change is acceptable. This is part of the general consensus that we should do more for animal welfare, identified in Chapter 1.

Monsters and myths

Not all our domestic animals are monsters: some of the worst ideas about genetic selection and modification are myths. Indeed, there are areas where genetic change has brought major advantages to animal welfare and may yet bring more.[21] Susceptibility to certain diseases has been reduced by selection, and while we said earlier that attempts to make animals resistant to disease by genetic engineering had not yet been very successful, there may be progress here too. As one example, scientists in Australia are attempting to modify sheep so that they produce insecticide in their skin.[36] This would benefit farmers in two ways, reducing both their expenditure on pesticides and the risk to their health from sheep dipping. In addition, it could be much more effective than chemicals in preventing the major suffering that sheep endure from blowflies, lice and other parasites, or from alternative control methods such as tail docking.

However, there are some monsters around on our farms. Some of the changes produced by genetic selection – in growth rate, in egg and milk production – have gone too far. It is possible that the suffering produced can be alleviated by other genetic changes, or by advances in our housing and husbandry of these animals, and investigation of these possibilities should be seen as urgent. But if these problems cannot be alleviated quickly, then such selection should now be stopped and in some cases reversed.

There are also monster mice. They have undoubtedly contributed to human medicine, but it is not clear how much, and many articles extolling the benefits of genetic engineering in mice do not even mention the welfare of the mice concerned.[37] More effort must be made in future to balance the suffering of these animals against the benefits produced. When attention is given to animal welfare it is hard to avoid the conclusion that such work should be reduced rather than increased.

Conclusions

- Few species of animals have been domesticated. These were chosen for their suitability, so some of them have changed very little since domestication, but there are limits to their adaptability.
- Some features of some species have, however, been altered considerably by genetic selection. Many welfare problems have been produced, for example in farm animals bred for increased production of eggs, meat or milk.
- Some applications of genetic engineering do not cause suffering or may even reduce animal suffering. All genetic engineering is controversial, however, for people concerned about animal natures or animal rights.
- Suffering is caused by production of experimental animals, particularly mice, with diseases or other abnormalities, by genetic engineering or other techniques. In the vetting of such work, increased weight should be given to the animal suffering relative to the potential human benefits.
- Genetic techniques can also be used to improve animal welfare, or to avoid current management practices that cause welfare problems. Increased priority should be given to such applications. Some current selection programmes should be stopped or reversed.

References

1. Jarman, M.R. (1972) European deer economies and the advent of the Neolithic. In *Papers in Economic Prehistory* (ed. E.S. Higgs), pp. 125–49. Cambridge University Press, Cambridge.
2. Genesis, Chapter 30, *New International Translation of the Bible*. Hodder and Stoughton, London. (The quotation is abridged.)

3. Darwin, C. (1882) *The Variation of Animals and Plants Under Domestication.* 2nd edn. Murray, London.
4. Clutton-Brock, J. (1987) *A Natural History of Domesticated Mammals.* British Museum (Natural History), London.
5. Stolba, A. & Wood-Gush, D.G.M. (1989) The behaviour of pigs in a semi-natural environment. *Animal Production,* **48**, 419–25.
6. Kurz, J.C. & Marchinton, R.C. (1972) Radiotelemetry studies of feral pigs in South Carolina. *Journal of Wildlife Management,* **36**, 1240–8; Krosniunas, E.H. (1979) *Social facilitation and foraging behavior of the feral pig (Sus scrofa) on Santa-Cruz Island, California.* MA thesis, University of California, Davis.
7. Appleby, M.C., Hughes, B.O. & Elson, H.A. (1992) *Poultry Production Systems: Behaviour, Management and Welfare.* CAB International, Wallingford, UK.
8. Wood-Gush, D.G.M. (1959) A history of the domestic chicken from antiquity to the 19th century. *Poultry Science,* **38**, 321–6.
9. Hewson, P. (1986) Origin and development of the British poultry industry: the first hundred years. *British Poultry Science,* **27**, 525–39.
10. Anjum, A.D., Payne, L.N. & Appleby, E.C. (1989) Oviduct magnum tumours in the domestic fowl and their association with laying. *Veterinary Record,* **125**, 42–3.
11. Gregory, N.G. & Wilkins, L.J. (1989) Broken bones in domestic fowl: handling and processing damage in end-of-lay battery hens. *British Poultry Science,* **30**, 555–62.
12. Figure from Etches, R.J. (1996) *Reproduction in Poultry.* CAB International, Wallingford, UK.
13. Kestin, S.C., Knowles, T.G., Tinch, A.E. & Gregory, N.G. (1992) Prevalence of leg weakness in broiler chickens and its relationship to genotype. *Veterinary Record,* **131**, 190–4.
14. Webster, A.J.F. (1994) *Animal Welfare: A Cool Eye Towards Eden.* Blackwell, Oxford.
15. Savory, C.J., Maros, K. & Rutter, S.M. (1993) Assessment of hunger in growing broiler breeders in relation to a commercial restricted feeding programme. *Animal Welfare,* **2**, 131–52.
16. Photograph from the Roslin Institute.
17. FAWC (1992) *Report on the Welfare of Broiler Chickens.* Farm Animal Welfare Council, Tolworth.
18. Sørensen, P. (1989) Broiler selection and welfare. In *Proceedings, 3rd European Symposium on Poultry Welfare* (eds J.M. Faure & A.D. Mills), pp. 45–58. World Poultry Science Association, Tours, France.
19. Savory, C.J., Hocking, P.M., Mann, J.S. & Maxwell, M.H. (1996) Is broiler breeder welfare improved by using qualitative rather than quantitative food restriction to limit growth rate? *Animal Welfare,* **5**, 105–27.

20. Hocking, P.M. & Whitehead, C.C. (1990) Relationship between body fatness, ovarian structure and reproduction in mature females from different lines of genetically lean or fat broilers given different food allowances. *British Poultry Science*, **31**, 319–30.

21. Mills, A.D., Beilharz, R.G. & Hocking, P.M. (1997) Genetic selection. In *Animal Welfare* (ed. M.C. Appleby & B.O. Hughes), pp. 219–31. CAB International, Wallingford, UK.

22. Pursel, V.G., Pinkert, C.A., Miller, K.F., Bolt, D.J., Campbell, R.G., Palmiter, R.D., Brinster, R.L. & Hammer, R.E. (1989) Genetic engineering of livestock. *Science*, **244**, 1281–8.

23. Photograph by Paul Hosefros, *New York Times* Pictures.

24. Appleby, M.C. (1998) Genetic engineering, welfare and accountability. *Journal of Applied Animal Welfare Science*, **1**, 255–73.

25. van Reenen, C.G. & Blokhuis, H.J. (1993) Investigating welfare of dairy calves involved in genetic modification: problems and perspectives. *Livestock Production Science*, **36**, 81–90.

26. Carver, A.S., Dalrymple, M.A., Wright, G., Cottom, D.S., Reeves, D.B., Gibson, Y.H., Keenan, J.L., Barrass, J.D., Scott, A.R., Colman, A. & Garner, I. (1993) Transgenic livestock as bioreactors – stable expression of human α-1-antitrypsin by a flock of sheep. *Bio-Technology*, **11**, 1263–70.

27. White, D.J.G. & Wallwork, J. (1993) Xenografting: probability, possibility or pipe dream? *Lancet*, **342**, 879–81.

28. Wilmut, I., Schnieke, A.E., McWhir, J., Kind, A.J. & Campbell, K.H.S. (1997) Viable offspring derived from fetal and adult mammalian cells. *Nature*, **385**, 810–3.

29. Harvard University (1988) US Patent 4,736,866 (12 April).

30. Home Office (1998) *Statistics of Scientific Procedures on Living Animals, Great Britain 1997*. Her Majesty's Stationery Office, London.

31. Sandøe, P., Crisp, R. & Holtug, N. (1997) Ethics. In *Animal Welfare* (eds M.C. Appleby & B.O. Hughes), pp. 3–17. CAB International, Wallingford, UK.

32. Fox, M. (1990) Transgenic animals: ethical and animal welfare concerns. In *The Bio-Revolution: Cornucopia or Pandora's Box?* (eds P. Wheale & R. McNally), pp. 31–45. Pluto Press, London.

33. Cochlan, A. (1993) Pressure group broods over altered turkeys. *New Scientist*, 29th April, p. 9.

34. Reiss, M. & Straughan, R. (1996) *Improving Nature? The Science and Ethics of Genetic Engineering*. Cambridge University Press, Cambridge.

35. Rollin, B.E. (1995) *The Frankenstein Syndrome: Ethical and Social Issues in the Genetic Engineering of Animals*. Cambridge University Press, Cambridge.

36. Dayton, L. (1992) 'Self-dipping' sheep will poison parasites. *New Scientist*, 4th April, p. 19.

37. Betsholtz, C. (1997) The mouse as a genetic model organism. In *Transgenic Animals and Food Production* (ed. A. Nilsson), pp. 45–50. Royal Swedish Academy of Agriculture and Forestry, Stockholm.

Chapter 6
Home is where the heart is: Housing and environments

Preconceptions and contradictions

A couple of years ago I visited Taiwan and went round the zoo in the capital Taipei. There had been a concerted attempt to design and equip the enclosures to mimic natural environments: the water buffalo had a bamboo grove and the macaques had rock ledges and creepers. There were two striking exceptions. The pigs were in a square concrete pen; the keepers had just accepted the common preconception that a pig's natural environment is a pigsty. Many of the other enclosures – including that of the macaques – were only naturalistic above ground-level; the floors were bare and hosed down daily. This common zoo practice is also based on a preconception, that it is necessary to wash cages regularly to avoid infection, for all species including monkeys. Unfortunately this attempt to safeguard one aspect of welfare causes problems with other aspects. Macaques in the wild regularly spend time on the ground, searching for food, socializing and playing. Those kept in enclosures with wet concrete floors rarely do so, and their behaviour is severely constrained as a result.

Many decisions about animal housing and husbandry have been strongly affected by preconceptions in this way, and many have contradictory effects on welfare (as we saw briefly in Chapter 2). This chapter is concerned with problems like these and with attempts to avoid them.

In fact, the particular problem of hygiene *versus* natural flooring in monkey cages can readily be resolved, because in this case the preconception about the need for washing is simply wrong. Primatologist Arnold Chamove added woodchips as floor litter to the cages of eight different monkey species at Edinburgh Zoo.

He also encouraged them to rake through the litter by adding food:

> Aggressive behavior was reduced by a factor of 3 with woodchips and by almost 10 times with grain or mealworms added to the litter. All negative behavior decreased by a factor of over 5 when food was added to the woodchips. Time spent on the ground almost doubled with woodchips, and more than doubled when food items were added to it. These effects occur in monkeys of various ages ... In addition, there is no evidence that using woodchips presents a health hazard. As the litter matures, the woodchips become increasingly more inhibitory to bacterial survival. This self-sterilizing action makes it likely that the mere presence of an absorbent litter greatly reduces the probability of disease spread due to fecal contamination.[1]

As a result of this sort of work, many zoos are starting to use natural flooring such as woodchips or earth in monkey cages.

There are two main reasons why simple improvements of this sort in the housing of captive animals are relatively rare. The first is that making one change often has many diverse effects. Sometimes these are beneficial, as in the example just given, but sometimes they are damaging. One attempt to make cages more interesting for laboratory mice had to be abandoned because adding objects to the cages increased the territoriality and aggression of the males and was judged to do more harm than good.[2] As a rule, it is important to consider the whole environment, not just one feature of it. Secondly, there are of course other constraints. Making changes involves time, thought, effort and – doubtless most important – money.

To put it the other way round, many welfare problems of captive animals have evidently been caused by excessive consideration of human needs rather than those of the animals. The question is how to redress that imbalance.

We should emphasize again, as we did in discussion of genetic selection, that this imbalance cannot simply be described as selfishness on the part of the individual humans concerned (although those individuals may have special responsibilities, as emphasized in Chapter 1). Farmers do not generally make bigger profits from giving animals less space, when they are selling their products in a competitive market, because to be competitive they must continually pare profit margins to the minimum. Scientists do not make a profit from giving their mice smaller cages. The selfishness involved could more accurately be attributed to society as a whole. However, before we get into detailed discussion of the need for society-wide decisions on the housing and treatment of animals, we need to consider at more length the complex effects on welfare of housing design and other aspects of environmental variation.

Cry freedom

The relationship between welfare and environments is not simple. For a start, we have to bear in mind the diversity of opinion about welfare, discussed in Chapter 2. Thus, people who put most emphasis on animal natures, on natural conditions and natural behaviour sometimes say that animals should be given freedom, as if that were all that needs to be said. But other people more concerned with animal bodies – with health and reproduction, for example – point out that 'freedom' brings disadvantages as well as advantages.

The same problem applies to specific 'freedoms'. Recall the five freedoms outlined by the Farm Animal Welfare Council. Now consider the following, written by British politician Roy Hattersley reviewing a book on human rights:

> If (with Kant) we believe that the only inalienable right is freedom, and (like Hobbes and Spinoza) we define that ideal condition as the absence of restraint, all the rights arguments fall neatly into place. But once we begin to talk about "freedom to" as well as "freedom from", the issue becomes more complicated. For freedoms collide.[3]

Thus freedom to speak our minds collides with freedom of others not to be offended by our opinions. Yet this is a balancing act we must attempt, because we value free speech as well as freedom from prejudice.

Where do we start with animal environments? One useful approach is to distinguish between the physical environment, the social environment – whether animals are housed alone or with other members of their species – and the interactions between animals and humans. These aspects overlap, but the first two are considered below and the third in the following chapter.

Stone walls and iron bars

When Oscar Wilde said that 'Stone walls do not a prison make, nor iron bars a cage',[4] he meant that for humans it is the loss of freedom and the social stigma of prison that are important, not the physical environment as such. Animals may lack understanding of such things, but as we saw in Chapter 3 that doesn't necessarily mean that they suffer less: for example, they may also not understand that imprisonment is temporary. Furthermore, the physical environment is critical to animal welfare. It seems difficult to recapture the mindframe of those in the nineteenth century who took lions, gorillas, elephants from the wild and put them into tiny cages or concrete bearpits – until we realize that it is still happening. Pigs in a pigsty, mice in a square plastic cage, puppies in a shoebox and, indeed, some zoo animals, are still given conditions that can be seen, once the preconceptions are pointed out, to be astonishingly cramped and barren.

Cramped and barren. There are the two main points: the amount of space provided and the nature of that space. We shall explore these two points in relation to the best known example of cramped, barren housing – battery cages.

In developed countries, most hens laying eggs for sale are kept in battery cages. Hens in breeding flocks, laying eggs for hatching, are usually not kept in cages. Nor, incidentally, are broiler chickens, so the common phrase 'I don't eat battery chicken' is true but misconceived.

The commonest arrangement is to have groups of four or five in wire cages, and in the European Community the minimum size for cages is $450\,cm^2$ per bird.[5] People sometimes illustrate that by saying that it is equivalent to three-quarters of an A4 sheet of paper. Insofar as that conjures up the image of a cage 21 cm × 21 cm it is a slightly misleading image, because hens are not caged singly. However, it is not far wrong. Four hens can be kept in a cage the size of three sheets of paper. Most farms keep five birds in a cage 50 cm × 50 cm – the size of an armchair cushion.

Marian Dawkins, who researches animal behaviour and welfare in Oxford, took photographs of hens from above, using the type of bird most common in the UK (which are brown and lay brown eggs).[6] She found that even just standing still a hen occupied $475\,cm^2$, and to turn round or to preen its feathers it used about $1200\,cm^2$ (Fig. 6.1). The white birds used elsewhere in the world are slightly smaller, but it is also true that in many

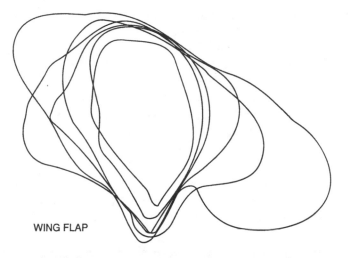

WING FLAP

Fig. 6.1 The space used for wing-flapping by an unrestricted hen. Successive outlines of birds were drawn from an overhead video picture, starting with the smallest outline when the bird was standing still.[6]

parts of the world – for example, in the USA – cages are even smaller than in Europe. So vast numbers of hens are unable even to stand without pressing against each other or overlapping. Turning round is difficult and they have to preen one at a time, rather than together as they do when given more space.

Furthermore, apart from the hens the cage is empty. It does not provide the environmental features necessary for the hens to peck, scratch, dustbathe or nest. To take nesting as an example, we know that a hen will walk a long way or do a great deal of work, every day, to find an appropriate place to lay her egg – a level or hollow place with some cover from predators.[7] Every day she is prevented from doing so and forced to lay the egg on a sloping floor in an open wire cage. There is widespread agreement with the Farm Animal Welfare Council's principle that animals should have freedom to express normal behaviour. There is less agreement on which specific behaviours should be provided for, but we have more evidence on the importance of nesting for hens than for any other behaviour in any other animal (apart from life-sustaining behaviour such as eating and drinking). Yet no provision is made for this behaviour in the battery cage.

Ban the battery cage? Unfortunately it isn't as simple as that. Hens have welfare problems in other housing systems too, which may seem even worse than those in batteries – as we shall see below. As an alternative approach, there have been projects in Edinburgh and elsewhere[8] on the possibility of increasing the size of cages and providing nest boxes, perches and dustbaths within them (Fig. 6.2). These 'enriched cages' reduce many of the welfare problems of batteries – although they don't remove them altogether. Meanwhile, at the time of writing the Commission of the European Communities is planning to increase minimum cage size to $800\,cm^2$ per bird, but not yet to require provision of facilities such as nest boxes.[9]*

In some cases barrenness *can* be reduced beneficially by a simple change, like addition of woodchips to the floor. Another scientist studying animal behaviour, Natalie Waran, added a

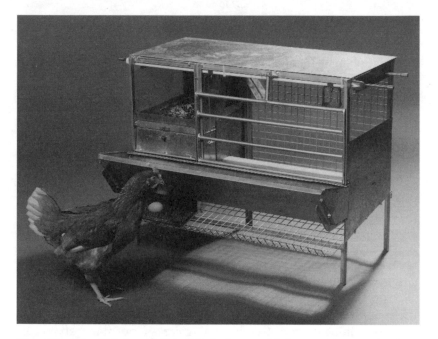

Fig. 6.2   The Edinburgh Modified Cage, which provides perch, dust bath (upper left) and nest box (lower left) for laying hens, as well as more space and height than conventional battery cages. This design is still experimental, but commercial development has begun.

---

* *Stop Press:* In June 1999, while this book was at the proof stage, the Commission strengthened its plans. Barren battery cages are now to be phased out in the EU and from 2012 all cages must be enriched.

simple partition to the pens of growing pigs, and found that it reduced aggression and increased growth rate (and hence profitability).[10] The young pigs were better able to escape from each other, by dodging behind the partition, and so fights were fewer and shorter than in normal, open pens. The point here, though, is that these changes were relevant to the animals concerned: they addressed specific problems that the animals had in their previous housing. In other cases, specific problems need more complex changes – such as the addition of nest boxes needed to allow hens to perform nesting behaviour in cages – or radical changes to the whole environment.

One phrase that is commonly used in this context is environmental enrichment. The concept is less than wholly satisfactory, for two reasons. First, it often starts from an extremely impoverished basis. When a rabbit is being kept in a cage too small for it to hop or stretch, addition of twigs for it to chew may be beneficial but could hardly be described as giving it a rich environment.

Second, the phrase more often refers to attempts to enrich the environment than to success. For example, a scientific paper that was published with the title 'Effects of enrichment and housing on cortisol response in juvenile rhesus monkeys'[11] did not actually find any such effects: the results of the study were negative. It would therefore better have been called 'Lack of effects of environmental *change* on cortisol response in juvenile rhesus monkeys'. Part of the problem is that the changes made are often irrelevant to the animals – as they were in this case.

However, increasing numbers of attempts at environmental enrichment are being made, and many seem to be beneficial. Some of the most successful are those concerned with methods of feeding, where the relevance to the animal is evident.

A major welfare problem for many animals in captivity is that they can eat their food very quickly, by contrast with the wild where they spend more than half their time looking for food and eating it. Their excess feeding behaviour is often expressed in strange, stereotyped behaviours such as the figure-of-eight pacing of polar bears (see Fig. 2.2). Work in Edinburgh has addressed this problem in pigs and horses.[12] A specially designed ball is filled with food; both pigs and horses quickly learn to push it around with their snout or muzzle, because every now and again some of the food drops out through a hole (Fig. 6.3). The animals spend more of their days foraging, as in the

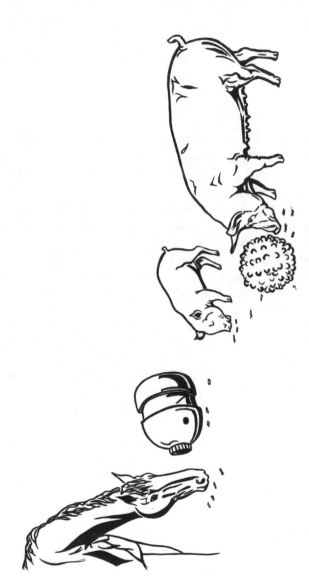

Fig. 6.3   The Equiball for horses and the Edinburgh Foodball for pigs both encourage animals to spend time foraging. When they push the ball around, small amounts of food occasionally drop out.

wild, and less stereotypic behaviour is seen. These foodballs are now being marketed, and it is telling that many more are selling for horses – where owners' criteria are not primarily commercial – than for pigs.

A sheep on its own

The physical environment is important, but we mustn't forget that a major part of the world for animals – just as it is for humans – is each other. First and foremost, we saw in Chapter 5 that one of the main factors in our choice of animals for domestication was that they lived in groups. Yet we keep many animals on their own: the sow in a farrowing crate, the rat in a cage, the dog left all day in the house.

Sheep are not often kept in isolation, but even with sheep the farmer may bring a ewe into the barn for treatment almost without thinking about it. Yet the New Zealand researcher on livestock behaviour and husbandry, Ron Kilgour, always said that sheep are such intensely social animals that 'A sheep on its own is not a sheep'. This importance of sociality was confirmed when Neil Baldock and Richard Sibly, in the UK, recorded heart rates of sheep as they were given various treatments.[13] When a single sheep was separated from the flock by a fence, she stayed calm and there was no effect on her heart rate, as long as she could see her companions. However, if the fence was solid she vocalized and tried to escape – indeed, two of the experimental animals succeeded in escaping – and her heart rate increased by 20 beats per minute. This treatment was more stressful than many of the others that the experimenters expected to be worse, such as handling by a human or being transported in a trailer.

We even condemn many companion animals to solitary confinement. It might seem that we keep them for themselves rather than for their monetary value, but the way we treat them shows that often we keep them more for our benefit than for theirs. Horses are social animals, yet most are kept in single stables, often without even being able to see another horse. Everyone who has seen two horses together knows their beautiful habit of mutual grooming – each nibbling the shoulders and neck of the other, cleaning and massaging the parts of the body that they cannot themselves reach (Fig. 6.4). Another fascinating study of heart rate showed that their hearts beat more slowly during this

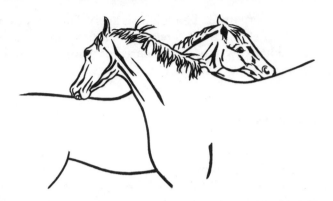

Fig. 6.4 Pairs of horses groom each other simultaneously, cleaning and massaging parts of the body that they cannot reach themselves.

grooming, suggesting that they are not only cleaning but also calming each other.[14]

Single housing in commercial farms or laboratories is another example of contradictory effects on welfare. One of the main reasons for it is to avoid aggression between animals. But there is obviously special pleading here. Certainly aggression can be a problem among pigs crowded in a bare pen. One particular reason is that a pig has no 'submission display' – no way of signalling to an aggressor that she submits, she accepts that the other is boss. Submission displays are well known in dogs and are also shown, for example, by cows. A submissive cow lowers her neck and lifts her chin, which lays her horns back on her neck and makes them less conspicuous. The only way a pig can show submission is by running away, which is impossible in a small pen. But aggression is less of a problem if pigs are given more space, or if they are given a varied or complex environment – as was shown by the experiment, described above, that provided a partition round which they could escape. As we said, avoiding problems involves time, thought, effort and money.

Apart from the physical conditions in which a group is housed, there are a number of major factors that affect social problems: stocking density, group size, group composition and mixing between individuals (Box 6.1). The influence of several of these can be illustrated in one example: the housing of laying hens in systems other than battery cages.

A major problem with all commercial housing systems other than cages for laying hens is that they involve large groups,

---

Box 6.1   Grouping of animals: important factors, illustrated in farm animals

Stocking density

High stocking density can lead directly to social problems, as in the example of aggression in pigs. Very high stocking density, as in battery cages, severely restricts behaviour.

Group size

Wild cattle live in groups of up to about 30, but domestic cattle may be kept in groups of several hundred. They cannot remember all the other individuals in the group and social interactions are complicated and protracted.

Group composition

Aggression is often more frequent in groups that consist of similar rather than varied individuals. Thus if piglets are matched for weight after weaning they fight more than if the group is diverse.

Mixing

Mixing new individuals together often causes problems and needs careful management – for example, allowing them to become acquainted through a fence before putting them in together.

---

typically of a thousand or more birds.[15] Chickens are descended from Jungle Fowl (Chapter 5), that live in groups of up to about 15 birds, and their social behaviour in these vast flocks is disrupted. Worst of all is that cannibalism is common: some birds peck others to death, often eating part of their flesh. We don't know exactly why they do this, but it is more common in large groups than small, at high stocking density than low, and in newly mixed groups than in stable flocks. It is also affected by the fact that the birds are in the uniform groups typical of commercial production and are all trying to do similar things – like laying in nest boxes – at the same time. The main way of preventing cannibalism is beak trimming – cutting off part of the birds' beaks. However, this is itself a serious welfare problem (Chapter 7).

This is still special pleading. It is possible to keep chickens without either putting them in cages or trimming their beaks, yet with a low risk of cannibalism: in small-scale farmyard flocks. But these are not commercially viable. In other words, many of the contradictory effects on welfare that we have been discussing throughout this chapter are avoidable in theory, but may not be avoidable in practice. In theory we could perhaps give ideal conditions to the zoo macaque, the pet horse, the farm chicken – while remembering that people will always disagree on precisely what those conditions would be like. In practice, any serious attempt to do so would probably mean that it was too expensive to keep zoo, pet or farm animals at all – and as we said in Chapter 4, that is an unsatisfactory conclusion. So what are we to do?

A dog is for life

The answer must involve compromise. Solutions do not have to be all-or-nothing – indeed, they cannot be all-or-nothing. In an ideal world it might be best neither to keep hens in cages nor to trim their beaks, but in the real world we can be confident that increasing the size of the cages and providing them with at least some facilities such as perches and nest boxes would have a real effect on welfare.

There is already compromise: both animals and humans receive benefit from our interactions (Chapter 4). However, as we also established in previous chapters, the compromise must shift further in the animals' favour, as we recognize our responsibility to do more for animal welfare. This is particularly apparent in intensive farming.

The point is made graphically in the slogan coined by animal charities to remind us of our responsibility for pets: A dog is for life, not just for Christmas (Fig. 6.5). The same applies to other animals too. Keeping animals involves commitment.

The compromise is shifting. Many or most zoos have changed almost beyond recognition in the last 10 years, in similar ways to the positive developments described at Taipei Zoo. Housing of farm and laboratory animals is changing much more slowly, partly because our financial and legal structures militate against change and complicate the decision processes. However, even on

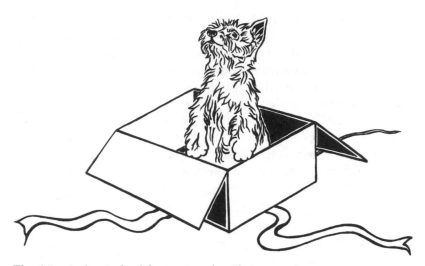

Fig. 6.5 A dog is for life, not just for Christmas.

farms and in laboratories there has been change: we have mentioned the increase in outdoor pig-keeping and there has been a similar increase in free-range poultry. Furthermore, regulations on animal housing are regularly introduced and more strictly enforced – although much remains to be done. Stalls and tethers for sows and crates for veal calves will soon be banned throughout the European Union.

In addition, there has been a change in attitude of the majority of people involved with animals that affects the ways in which animals are treated – their husbandry and handling, as well as their housing. Direct treatment of animals by humans is the subject of the next chapter.

Conclusions

- The physical environment has complex and contradictory effects on animal welfare, but the main problems for many animals kept by humans can be simply summarized: shortage of space and lack of facilities in the space that they have.
- Specific changes may improve welfare, particularly if they take the animals' biology into account. A biological approach is important in many aspects of environmental design, for example consideration of effects of experience over an animal's whole lifetime.

- Social animals should be kept socially, avoiding problems like aggression by appropriate environmental design and group composition rather than by solitary confinement.
- Decisions between housing systems – for example between battery cages and other systems for laying hens – are difficult and require compromises to be made. For animals kept commercially, compromise in the economic criteria applied will have to be enforced by legislation.
- There have been improvements over recent years in the ways in which many animals are kept, but many more changes are needed.

References

1. Chamove, A.S., Anderson, J.R., Morgan-Jones, S.C. & Jones, S.P. (1982) Deep woodchip litter: hygiene, feeding, and behavioural enhancement in eight primate species. *International Journal for the Study of Animal Problems*, **3**, 308–18.
2. McGregor, P.K. & Ayling, S.J. (1990) Varied cages result in more aggression in male CFLP mice. *Applied Animal Behaviour Science*, **26**, 277–81.
3. Hattersley, R. (1996) Collision of freedoms (review of N. Bobbio *The Age of Rights* (1996, Polity)). *Guardian Weekly*, 25th February.
4. Wilde, O. (1898) *The Ballad of Reading Gaol*. 4th edn. Smithers, London.
5. Commission of the European Communities (1986) Council Directive 86/113/EEC: Welfare of Battery Hens. *Official Journal of the European Communities (L 95)*, **29**, 45–9.
6. Dawkins, M.S. & Hardie, S. (1989) Space needs of laying hens. *British Poultry Science*, **30**, 413–6; figure from Dawkins, M.S. & Nicol, C.J. (1989) No room for manoeuvre. *New Scientist*, 16th September, 44–6.
7. Appleby, M.C. (1993) Should cages for laying hens be banned or modified? *Animal Welfare*, **2**, 67–80.
8. Appleby, M.C. & Hughes, B.O. (1995) The Edinburgh Modified Cage for laying hens. *British Poultry Science*, **36**, 707–18; Sherwin, C.M. (1994) *Modified Cages for Laying Hens*. Universities Federation for Animal Welfare, Potters Bar, UK.
9. Commission of the European Communities (1998) *Proposal for a Council Directive laying down minimum standards for the protection of laying hens kept in various systems of rearing*. COM (98). Commission of the European Communities, Brussels.
10. Waran, N.K. & Broom, D.M. (1993) The influence of a barrier on the behaviour and growth of early-weaned piglets. *Animal Production*, **56**, 115–9.

11. Schapiro, S.J., Bloomsmith, M.A., Kessel, A.L. & Shively, C.A. (1993) Effects of enrichment and housing on cortisol response in juvenile rhesus monkeys. *Applied Animal Behaviour Science*, **37**, 251–63.
12. Young, R.J., Carruthers, J. & Lawrence, A.B. (1994) The effect of a foraging device (The 'Edinburgh Foodball') on the behaviour of pigs. *Applied Animal Behaviour Science*, **39**, 237–47; Winskill, L.C., Waran, N.K. & Young, R.J. (1996) The effect of a foraging device (a modified 'Edinburgh Foodball') on the behaviour of the stabled horse. *Applied Animal Behaviour Science*, **48**, 25–35.
13. Baldock, N.M. & Sibly, R.M. (1990) Effects of handling and transportation on the heart rate and behaviour of sheep. *Applied Animal Behaviour Science*, **28**, 15–39.
14. Feh, C. & de Mazieres, J. (1993) Grooming at a preferred grooming site reduces heart rate in horses. *Animal Behaviour*, **46**, 1191–4.
15. Appleby, M.C., Hughes, B.O. & Elson, H.A. (1992) *Poultry Production Systems: Behaviour, Management and Welfare*. CAB International, Wallingford, UK.

Chapter 7
Give and take: Animal treatment

Fair exchange?

A piglet is born on the farm. The farmer has planned his birth and arranged for it to happen: she has given him life. She fattens him, then sends him to the abattoir: she takes his life away again. Is this a fair exchange?

No, because it is not just a question of what we do, but of how we do it. The young pig is fed and watered, but he spends his life in cramped, barren conditions – as discussed in Chapter 6 – and other aspects of the way he is treated may also be less than fair.

Farmers are not wantonly cruel. Most of those who rear animals do so because they like animals, and most show a fair degree of enlightened self-interest. A piglet treated badly by the farmer may die or grow more slowly: in many respects good treatment of animals benefits both the animals and the farmer. But there is an important exception to this rule. The farmer is concerned with animals *as a group*. Her main criterion is not the growth rate of this particular piglet and the profit she can gain from him; it is the performance of her whole pig unit and the economic balance sheet of her whole herd. So if she finds that rearing piglets in the dark, say, allows her to keep more in the same pen – because it reduces activity – then she may well do so. The growth rate of each piglet may actually be less, but the total profit from the pen will be more.

Again there is an imbalance. Farmers and other people involved with the economics of animal use are concerned with the health and welfare of the animals, but their primary concern is with group performance. From the animals' perspective, it is the individuals that matter.

Bernard Rollin describes a case in Canada where a vet

inspecting a large pig farm noticed a sow with a broken leg and was told they planned to keep her until she farrowed, then shoot her. This would be illegal in many countries. 'When he offered at least to splint the leg at cost, he was told that the operation [i.e. the farm] could not afford to expend the manpower which would be entailed by separating the sow and caring for her'.[1] Let us hope such extreme cases are rare, but the broiler chickens with leg problems (Chapter 4) are not so very different from that sow.

Animals reared only for meat, such as pigs and broilers, are in a category of their own among captive animals, because we gain little from them while they are alive. With other animals under our control the give and take might be expected to take into account the fact that what we gain from them we gain during their lives. We give life and sustenance to the pet dog, the laboratory mouse, the dairy cow. We take companionship, research results, milk. Do we look after them better than meat animals because these 'outputs' are long- rather than short-term? The answer, unfortunately, is no. Just as the pig and the broiler may yield an acceptable amount of meat despite less than ideal treatment, so the dog may keep her master company even if he kicks her.

What about wild animals? From some wild animals we simply take their lives, for food. Others we hunt for sport before we kill them. What do we give them? Maybe we give them conservation: a safeguarding of the opportunities of being born and living a reasonable life. Is this a fair exchange? How do we actually treat animals, in all these categories?

Open all hours

Life is a life sentence. It goes on for animals – as it does for us – 24 hours a day, 365 days a year, year after year for a lifetime.

Not many people kick their dogs, but many people ignore them, for as much as 23 hours a day. Many dogs are left alone for much of the time – in the house during the day, downstairs at night. This is perhaps even more true for horses. These are highly social animals, yet they are often kept alone and visited only once a day for feeding. We present such animals with a major problem: how to fill the rest of their time. This is the opposite problem to that faced by many wild animals, who have too few hours in the day to find food and their other needs. Furthermore, there are two factors that make the situation worse for many captive animals. First, as already emphasized, many are kept in barren conditions – the dog kennel, the laboratory cage, the circus menagerie. The worst welfare problem for many laboratory mice and circus elephants is what happens to them, not when they are being used – in the experiment or in the circus show – but when they are not. Secondly, many are kept hungry. This applies to some extent to pets such as dogs and zoo animals such as the big cats. It applies to an even greater extent to certain farm animals, particularly sows (Chapter 2) and the parents of broiler chickens (Chapter 5). These animals are not only hungry, they are also prevented from doing anything constructive about it, and this combination causes distress.[2] So in assessing our treatment of animals, we must consider not just the times that we see them but the whole of the day and night.

A similar argument applies at the next level up: we must take into account the effect on animals of day by day variation or the lack of it. In some cases we only see animals in good conditions. As we have seen (Chapter 2), people often have a rosy view of life in the wild, because they only see wild animals on sunny days, not when it is cold and wet. Sometimes they unwittingly make the situation worse. People enjoy feeding swans and ducks on public ponds, and doubtless intend to help the birds as well, but understandably they make many more visits in good weather than bad. The result is that waterfowl gather in such places (Fig. 7.1), but then run short of food on the very days when they need it most.[3]

Conversely, captive animals often have too little variation from day to day throughout the year. One advantage of bad days is that they make the other days good by contrast. Animals may be ill-equipped to deal with a world in which food is always available and it's neither too hot nor too cold – in which nothing unusual ever happens. Zoo managers have begun to learn this lesson. Until recently most zoo animals were fed on a rigid daily schedule, with the same amount at the same time day after day, in complete contrast to their unpredictable food supplies in the wild. Now it is increasingly common for big cats, for example, to be fed variable amounts at variable times – including some days with nothing at all. They no longer show the stereotyped pacing that used to occur before the regular feeding time, and they are more active and varied in their behaviour.

Of course, the lives of most animals go beyond days and months into years or decades. How we treat them has long-term

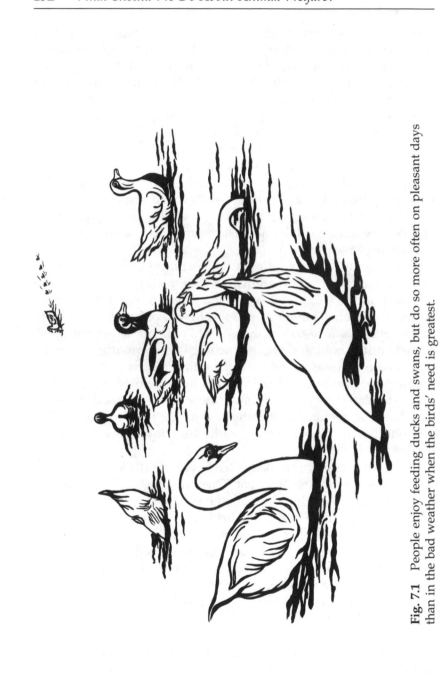

Fig. 7.1 People enjoy feeding ducks and swans, but do so more often on pleasant days than in the bad weather when the birds' need is greatest.

as well as short-term effects. This is particularly important because many problems are irreversible: they can be prevented but not cured. For example, horses in loose boxes frequently show crib biting: mouthing or biting the hay rack or the door stereotypically for long periods of time (Fig. 7.2).

We now know that, as with big cats, this is largely a reaction to the fact that because they are kept indoors and fed on food pellets, they cannot carry out their natural foraging behaviour. Unfortunately giving them hay or moving them to a field rarely helps once this behaviour is established: it has become pathological, and they simply shift to biting the fence round the field.[4] To avoid the behaviour we must feed horses throughout their lives in more appropriate ways (Chapter 6).

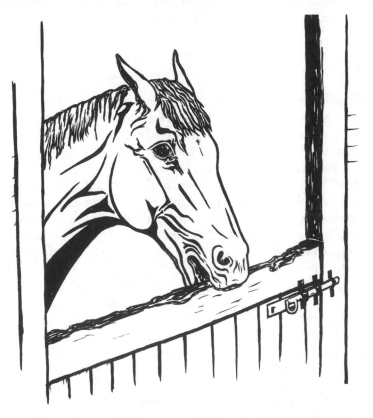

Fig. 7.2 Horses kept on their own and fed on food pellets often develop crib biting: mouthing or biting the hay rack or the door for long periods. Both their social and their foraging behaviour are strongly restricted in these conditions.

Solving such long-term problems is often difficult, because many factors are involved. We mentioned in Chapter 6 that hens are sometimes cannibalistic, and they also often peck at and remove each other's feathers. Many studies have suggested that rearing conditions are important – for example, that the tendency of chicks to peck at feathers is increased by a lack of other things to peck. However, there are so many other factors involved (such as group size), and so many other pressures on commercial management, and it is so difficult and expensive to set up experiments on a commercial scale, that definitive recommendations on rearing techniques to reduce this problem are elusive.[5]

The search for such definitive recommendations must continue, however, in many areas of animal management. Welfare cannot be assessed or improved from a snapshot: it involves a documentary of the animal's life story.

Day by day

That documentary includes both routine and one-off events. Routine events include milking and cleaning, exercising and working. One of the most fundamental routines is the fact that we turn the lights on and off. We get so used to living with a light switch ourselves that we forget it's unnatural – and that whereas we have control of the switch our animals don't. In fact animals are remarkably adaptable to variable light regimes. I sometimes feel guilty about giving my cats an extremely variable pattern of lighting in the evening, but they don't seem to notice – they sleep on, or sit in wakeful watchfulness, regardless. Similarly chickens are sometimes kept in intermittent light: they may be given a night of 10 hours, then alternating 2-hour periods of light and dark for the rest of the 24 hours, because they digest their food more efficiently on this system.[5] It seems a bizarre way to treat animals, but again they quickly adapt. They eat and rest alternately anyway, and under this regime they are constrained to do so in 2-hour bursts.

There is no evidence of suffering in these cases, but it is worth remembering that suffering is not the only criterion for poor welfare. Some people emphasize that animals should be kept in conditions that are as natural as possible – that they should be treated as animals, not as machines (Chapter 2) – and intermittent lighting is certainly not natural. Sometimes, indeed, an intuition that unnaturalness is wrong turns out to be supported by the existence of problems for animal feelings and functioning (for animal minds and bodies, as well as natures). This applies, for example, to another aspect of artificial lighting – the fact that changes between light and dark are usually abrupt. Laboratory rabbits usually have lights of this sort, controlled by a time clock, yet in the wild they restrict most of their behaviour to periods of twilight and are inactive in either bright light or complete darkness. It is now recommended that laboratory lighting should change more gradually at 'dusk' and 'dawn' and remain dim rather than completely dark in between,[6] but this is so far rare in laboratories.

Undoubtedly the most pervasive routine treatment that we impose on animals is feeding. We have already discussed many of the problems that arise from restriction of either food quantity or feeding time, and problems also come from feeding methods. For example, hens in battery cages are given 10 cm of food trough each.[5] They try to eat at the same time but they are wider than 10cm so they can't.

Some problems can be reduced quite easily once we put our minds to it. Thus the stereotypic pacing of polar bears in zoos happens before feeding. It seems that it happens because their natural behaviour involves spending a long time hunting or searching for food before eating, and when they are given a single rapidly-eaten meal at a predictable time that activity is redirected into the action of pacing. Solution: feed them first thing in the morning.[7] Obvious in retrospect, this simple measure has reduced the distressing pacing of many zoo bears. Another measure that helps is to require them to work for their food. In Copenhagen Zoo the polar bears are given fish frozen into blocks of ice.[8] It takes them a lot of time and ingenuity to break open the blocks to get at the fish.

Feeding is one area where contradictory effects on welfare are common. Food restriction causes hunger which is a major welfare problem, but giving animals as much food as they could eat would cause other problems such as obesity. Sometimes this dilemma is of our making – as with the parents of broiler chickens that we have selected for appetite (Chapter 5). But that is not always true: lions will also overeat given the chance. Another contradiction occurs in the feeding of laying hens. These birds prefer distinct pieces of food to small particles. However, in commercial conditions they are fed mash rather than pellets, because this takes them longer to eat and reduces the problem of feather pecking discussed above.[5]

Obviously it is impossible to generalize about the best feeding methods for all animals, but perhaps two principles are useful. Firstly, feeding is critically important:

> It is perhaps not accidental that in most existing codes of recommendations for the welfare of animals [including FAWC's five freedoms: Chapter 2] 'freedom from hunger and thirst' features as the first requirement that has to be satisfied.[9]

An army marches on its stomach, as Napoleon said, and so do most animals.

Secondly, two factors that are important in feeding are *control* and *predictability*. Control is always an advantage. A wild boar may get less to eat than a commercial sow, but still does not show stereotypic behaviour. This is because he can do something constructive about his hunger: he can search for food with some prospect of finding it. He is at least to some extent in control of his own life.

Predictability is sometimes a disadvantage, as with the big cats in zoos, discussed above. However, it is an advantage in browsing and grazing species of animals when food is restricted. The commercial sow kept on a limited ration shows even worse stereotypies if her meal does not arrive at its usual time.

In fact control and predictability (or conversely variability) are important in many other areas of animals' lives as well. This can be clearly demonstrated with one other type of event that is routine in some animals' lives: blood sampling and injections. For many years all laboratory and zoo primates were physically restrained for such procedures. However, it was recently realized – and it is another idea that seems obvious with hindsight – that they can be trained to co-operate just as easily as a child can. Rewarded with food after each injection, a chimpanzee will soon put her arm out through the bars for the next one. It is questionable whether laboratory work on chimpanzees should be allowed at all, but injections are needed in zoos too, and if they have to happen it is better that the animal should be in control of the situation rather than having to be held down.

Once in a lifetime

Lack of predictability is also a major factor in many one-off treatments of animals. The treatments are one-off for the animals, that is, but of course many such treatments are routine for the people concerned. This is one reason why little attention has often been given to effects on the animals.

You've just bought a young horse and you're in a hurry to get him home, but he's reluctant to climb the ramp into the horse box. You don't have this problem with any of your other horses, so you and the sellers use carrot and stick, encouraging him from the front and shoving from the back. Eventually he's in, but he's panting and staring and you can feel his heart racing as he leans against you. Why wouldn't he be scared of entering a dark box he's never seen before? With a bit more foresight the sellers could have parked a horse box in his paddock for a few days before-hand and fed him on the ramp or even inside. With experience, horses baulk less during loading.[10]

Many animals are transported only once – or only a limited number of times at long intervals and in different circumstances each time. Of course it's not just unfamiliarity that is at issue in our treatment of animals. In the case of transport, the actual conditions in which animals are transported are important – yet we often do not put such knowledge into practice for reasons of cost or convenience or tradition. Horses are more comfortable in a horse box if they face backwards, because they find it easier to brace themselves in that position,[11] but in practice this demands a box with two doors and ramps so that they can be loaded from the front – and such expensive boxes are still rare.

Among the other, multifarious things people do to animals, two categories will be considered here: mutilations and experi-mentation.

The term 'mutilation' is increasingly used for removal or alteration of parts of animals' bodies, 'calling a spade a spade'. Not surprisingly, the term is usually avoided by the people responsible. This is partly because in many cases it can be argued that the procedure is necessary, and the term 'mutilation' is unequivocally pejorative, but the point about terminology here is that it does colour the picture. For example, removal of part of hens' beaks used to be called debeaking. That was inaccurate, because not all the beak is removed. It is now usually called beak trimming. That is potentially misleading, because it sounds like hoof trimming or nail trimming, whereas in this case not just the horny beak is cut but the underlying tissue as well. The foremost authority on this procedure, Dr Mike Gentle of the Roslin Institute near Edinburgh, calls it partial beak amputation. That is accurate.

Beak trimming is objectionable for two main reasons. Firstly, as with any amputation, there is strong evidence that it causes pain.[12] Secondly, it removes the bird's second-most important sense organ (after the eyes), the touch-sensitive tip of the beak. However, it reduces aggression, feather pecking and cannibalism among hens (see above and Chapter 6) – because after trimming the beak is blunter and is generally used less. The combination of these effects means that it is difficult to decide whether to trim birds' beaks. If their beaks are trimmed they suffer pain and sensory deprivation, perhaps unnecessarily. If not, they are at risk of an outbreak of even more painful feather pecking, cannibalism or both. The Farm Animal Welfare Council comments as follows in a report on the welfare of laying hens:

> We consider that the mutilation of all livestock is undesirable and continue to regard beak trimming as a major welfare insult. We do, however, recognise that in some systems such procedures may currently be necessary. Where the operation is performed correctly, it can help to avoid worse problems. Nonetheless, the ultimate aim should be the avoidance of beak trimming.[13]

The vital point is that although the procedure is 'currently necessary' and routine – it is performed on millions of chicks each year – this should not prevent us from trying firstly to minimize the welfare problem and secondly to prevent it altogether. On the first count, Mike Gentle has recently shown that if birds' beaks must be trimmed, it is better to do it shortly after hatching than later. At a young age they probably suffer short-term pain but this soon passes, whereas later amputation seems to cause long-term phantom stump pain, similar to that from crude amputations in humans.[14] Fortunately most commercial beak trimming is now done soon after hatching and the more serious operation needed for older birds is now rare. On the second count, there has been some progress in the USA on selecting birds that do not peck each other, even with intact beaks.[15] Further work on such selection should be a priority in the poultry industry.

There are other mutilations that involve similar dilemmas. Many lambs have their tails docked, because otherwise they later get covered with dung and are liable to insect attack. We now know, though, that the usual method of putting a tight rubber ring on the tail so that it dies and drops off is almost certainly acutely painful.[16] Better methods should be used, possibly including anaesthetic.

There are yet other mutilations, however, not involving such dilemmas, that are done for cosmetic reasons, such as whisker-trimming of dogs to conform with the standards expected at dog shows. Such intrusions on an animal's body, painful or not, are unwarranted. They are on the decline and should be phased out altogether.

Animal experiments are also on the decline. The decline is uneven, with work in some areas such as genetic engineering on the increase (Chapter 5), but real. The number of animals used each year in experiments licensed by the UK Home Office fell by half from 5.5 million in the mid-1970s to 2.6 million in 1997[17] and there have been similar decreases in other European countries.[18] There are also changes in the type of animals used: for example, much testing of potentially toxic compounds is now done on fish rather than mammals, and while this is not an unequivocal gain in welfare terms (Chapter 3) most people would agree that it is a gain. In addition, development of alternative techniques such as testing toxicity on cell cultures is progressing.

In brief, the principle of the three Rs has become widespread, that there should be *replacement*, *reduction* and *refinement* of the use of animals in experiments. To give one example, it used to be a legal requirement that cosmetics or their constituents were tested on animals before being marketed to check whether they caused skin or eye irritation. It still is required in some countries. However, such tests have been phased out in some countries such as the UK and Germany, and have been considerably reduced in others. This is for several reasons: results of tests can now be exchanged between countries; testing may only be necessary if there are new constituents; more is known about which constituents are likely to be irritant and so these can be avoided without testing. Lastly, the procedure now used – in those countries where it is used at all – is to test only one animal at a time. If the first animal shows irritation, no others are tested, and the test on that one is terminated immediately. Photographs of animals with suppurating eyes, displayed by campaigners against such tests, are certainly not typical and probably out of date. There is nothing to be gained by taking tests as far as that.[19] Furthermore, while it is possible that in past decades the scientists and technicians involved used to be uncaring about their animals, their views have changed now.

One of the problems is that the whole subject is so emotive. In a book called *The Cruel Deception: The Use of Animals in Medical Research*,[20] Robert Sharpe listed some of the experiments carried out in the UK and USA in the early 1980s. Many certainly caused gross animal suffering – and in the UK would not have been possible after 1986 when the *Animal (Scientific Procedures) Act* became law, but his list also included the following:

> 1983: Chemical Defence scientists publish experiments in which rhesus monkeys are anaesthetized and shot in the head with high velocity missiles.

This sounds unpleasant, and it is certainly questionable whether it should have been done. Yet the experimental procedure itself did not apparently cause major problems for welfare, because the animals were unconscious. Failure to make this sort of distinction has often impeded discussion about animal experiments.

The situation is improving in animal experimentation, with direct government oversight in some countries and institutional animal care and use committees (IACUCs) mandatory in others. In the USA, IACUCs were established in 1985 following publicity about exactly the sort of cases highlighted by Sharpe.[20]

And yet, and yet ... These changes have not gone far enough. As we said in Chapter 5, more weight should be given to animal suffering when experimental plans are vetted. One of the problems is that in most countries there is no information available on what is actually done or on how the weighing was carried out. As the RSPCA comments, concerning the UK's *Animal (Scientific Procedures) Act*:

> Only a limited amount of information is published in the annual statistics. There is no way of finding out either the costs or benefits, how the research was justified when the project was licensed, or how well the Act is administered or implemented. It is not possible to tell which new substances are

being developed and tested or the extent to which they are actually needed or may be of benefit. Neither is it possible to tell what is actually done to animals in any of the procedures listed, whether this causes suffering and if so how much.[21]

For example, the *Home Office Statistics*[17] tell us that 50% of procedures done under the *Animal (Scientific Procedures) Act* in 1997 were for 'protection of man, animals or the environment' or were 'applied studies, for veterinary or human medicine'. The remainder were for 'fundamental biological research', 'breeding' or other purposes. Yet we are not told how many of this remainder caused animal suffering, or how decisions were made about whether this was justified.

Some people who support animal rights think that no experiments causing animal suffering are ever justifiable. However, they are a small minority, partly because it is difficult to maintain such an absolutist position consistently with regard to all the decisions that have to be taken about animals (Chapter 1). But on the other hand, few people think that *all* types of experiments can be justified, even if they might lead to considerable benefit. The majority of people adopt a mixed view, which has been well expressed by the Banner Committee. This was set up by the UK government to consider the ethics of breeding techniques for farm animals, but its conclusions apply more widely:

a) Harms of a certain degree and kind ought under no circumstances to be inflicted on an animal.
b) Any harm to an animal, even if not absolutely impermissible, nonetheless requires justification and must be outweighed by the good which is realistically sought in so treating it.
c) Any harm which is justified by the second principle ought, however, to be minimized as far as is reasonably possible.[22]

Indeed, these conclusions apply to all our treatment of animals. What we do to animals requires more thought, more justification – and more moderation – than we have used hitherto.

To see ourselves as others see us

This need for consideration extends not just to what we do and the way that we do it, but to the fact that it is we who are doing it.

Humans are a profoundly important part of animals' environments. For a start, do they see us as parents or predators, food or rivals? You pick up a hamster to stroke (Fig. 7.3). He bites you. Why are you surprised? Yet the relationship between animals and humans is often complex, often positive. Many hamsters and other pets do appear to enjoy being stroked. Doubtless we are mimicking the grooming that they received from their parents when they were younger. Laboratory rats will press a lever repeatedly to earn the reward of being petted by a human.[23]

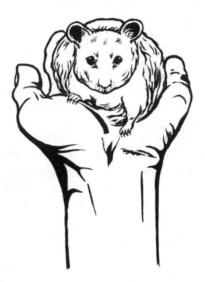

Fig. 7.3   Does a hamster see you as a parent or as a predator?

Failure to understand the importance of such relationships has often caused major problems. For example, early in the twentieth century some zoos stopped training their elephants, because the public mood had shifted away from gawping at performing animals towards admiring what it saw as the wild and natural: elephant rides were out of fashion. The change was disastrous. As soon as they were half-grown the elephants were completely unmanageable. No-one could approach them without extreme caution and they caused a lot of damage, including to themselves. Several had to be shot. If elephants are to live in captivity, it is far better both for them and their keepers if they are socialized to humans. What is more, a group of elephants gives every appearance of enjoying its interactions with a keeper, a hose and a brush.

People's failure to train their dogs properly is generally a mixture of laziness and ignorance, yet it has huge effects on their lives. A neighbour of ours is currently training her dog, unwittingly but systematically, to bark in the garden. Every time he barks she gives him a biscuit to shut him up. Not surprisingly, he does it again before long. Where will it end? With him being shut in the house all day, or de-barked surgically?

Perhaps surprisingly, there has been more careful research done on the relationship of farm animals to humans than that of pets – because there are a lot more farm animals in similar situations whereas every pet is unique, and because with farm animals there are economics involved. Some of the most important work has been done by Paul Hemsworth in Australia. One of his early results,[24] that set the theme for all his subsequent work, came when he found that pig farms with generally similar management nevertheless varied in productivity. Some had piglets who grew faster, and sows who had larger litters, than others. On the more productive farms, pigs were less frightened of people: if he climbed into a pen full of pigs they would approach him rather than trying to get away. The explanation for both aspects of variation was in the behaviour of the stockmen. On some farms the pigmen were rough with their pigs, continually shoving and slapping them. Blood tests showed that these pigs became stressed, and this depressed their growth and reproduction. Not surprisingly, they also became fearful of humans. On other farms, though, the stockmen were fond of their pigs: they gave them names, talked to them and handled them gently. These pigs were not stressed, they produced well and they readily approached people.

Hemsworth has proceeded to show that people working with stock can be trained to have a positive attitude to animals and that this improves their stockmanship. This then has positive effects on both animal production and animal welfare[25] – which appeals, as we said before, to the enlightened self-interest of the farmers.

Furthermore, the workers doubtless enjoy their job more if they are co-operating with their animals rather than fighting them. Indeed, even when pigs or hens are being their most annoying, and going in every direction except the one you want, losing your temper with them usually makes herding them slower rather than faster – and makes you feel worse too.

One major factor that affects the attitude and behaviour of

workers to animals is the design of housing and other systems, yet such design has generally given far too little attention to the comfort, convenience and enjoyment of the people who will be using them. In systems that are uncomfortable and inefficient to operate, it is not surprising if workers become impatient and frustrated, and treat animals roughly. I saw one farm worker loading pigs into a truck. The ramp didn't have proper gates at the side, so one pig slipped off. Rather than let it run off, or risk all the others escaping too, he grabbed it by the tail and one ear and heaved it back onto the truck. Similarly, a colleague watched operations at an ill-designed slaughter house, where the sheep regularly baulked at a sharp turn in a corridor.[26] The workers had to heave every single sheep round the corner – and would probably have been rougher if he hadn't been watching.

Would you want to work in a slaughterhouse? If you had to, would you want to spend every working day of your life wrestling sheep, rather than have them moving smoothly through a well-designed system? If you had to do *that*, would you go on being gentle with every sheep?

Past, present and future

It sometimes seems that although much has been said about welfare over the last 30 years there has not been much actual improvement: experiments on laboratory animals and mutilation of farm animals still continue. However, this impression is misleading. Firstly, and perhaps most importantly, there has been a change in the attitude of the majority of people involved with animals, at least in developed countries (less developed countries will be discussed in Chapter 9). This has led to many improvements in husbandry, which is crucial to welfare. Secondly, there have been innumerable changes which are relatively inconspicuous but nevertheless important: stronger enforcement of legislation, reductions in the numbers of experimental animals used, phasing out of harmful procedures, development of alternatives for animal use in school, college and university teaching. Thirdly, there have been some major changes. In relation to specific treatments of animals, perhaps the most important, as emphasized above, is that animal experimentation in many countries is now overseen by institutional animal care and use committees, and carried out with the three Rs – reduction, refinement and replacement – in mind.

Yet there are other ways of treating animals governed more by tradition than by current attitudes. Hunting is one such area. Indeed, one of the major arguments made in favour of hunting is that if it hadn't been for hunting, there would have been less conservation of the areas where the hunted species live and many of them would no longer exist. That may be true, but it doesn't follow that it has to be true in future: there is now, of course, increased support for conservation as well as for better animal treatment.

The most controversial form of hunting is pursuit of mammals – particularly deer and foxes – with dogs and horses. There is certainly tradition involved here. As Pat Bateson points out in his report on deer hunting:

> To many people, witnessing a hunt is to feel part of English history and the sight of the full field of horses and hounds is both beautiful and thrilling. The field-craft of the huntsmen is remarkable and the skill of the hounds marvellous to watch.[27]

Furthermore, many of those involved believed that the study would vindicate them: that running from a predator was a normal part of a deer's life and so not especially harmful. That was probably why they co-operated with Bateson and his assistant. However, Bateson does quote one man who was clearly aware of the issues:

> One farmer, who has been an ardent stag hunter all his life, said to us 'If your report goes against us, then perhaps we shouldn't be doing what we're doing'.

The report did go against them: it showed that hunting was extremely stressful to the deer (Chapter 4). Deer hunting is now banned on National Trust land in England, and fox hunting is under increasing pressure.

Other treatments of animals are undergoing more rapid change. A development that is having an impact on treatment of farm animals – and will have more impact in future – is automation. To give just one example, the development of automatic milking machines is proceeding rapidly.[28] Such a machine allows each cow to enter at a time of her choosing, recognizes her by microchip, calls up its memory of the shape of her udder and then uses a robotic arm to put the teat cups in place for milking. There may be advantages and disadvantages for welfare. Cows will be able to visit the machine several times each day and relieve the pressure on udders otherwise distended by selection for milk production. Low ranking animals will no longer be pushed into the parlour between high rankers they'd prefer to avoid. But on the other hand, the fact that cows will be handled less frequently by humans will mean that those procedures for which they still have to be handled – such as foot trimming – will be more stressful.

Advocates of automation suggest that farmers will spend more time looking after animals:

> [It] will eliminate many hazardous, tedious or unpleasant chores undertaken by farmers. They, in turn, will be freed for those tasks for which man is uniquely suited.[29]

The likelihood of course is that instead, fewer people will be employed to look after the animals, and the animals will in consequence be less well looked after.

There are gains and losses in treatment of animals, both for humans and for the animals concerned. There is give and take, and in many cases that give and take cannot be said to constitute fair exchange. In some cases, perhaps, the exchange is getting fairer, but there's still a lot of room for improvement.

Conclusions

- For animals in our control, welfare must be considered 24 hours a day, year after year, not just at the times that we are using them or interacting with them.
- Routine treatments have major impacts on animals. One important factor here is the extent to which an animal is in control of its own life. Another is predictability of treatments, which is an advantage in some circumstances (such as feeding, when food is restricted), but a disadvantage in others (variability in feeding time is beneficial for well-fed animals).
- Treatments that are routine for the people performing them – though not for the animals concerned – have sometimes received insufficient scrutiny. More effort should be put into avoiding mutilation of animals, and experiments on animals should be subjected to a broad ethical scrutiny, not just a utilitarian cost–benefit analysis.
- Humans are themselves an important part of animals'

environments, and interactions with animals are often critical for welfare. These can be improved both by encouraging the development of appropriate attitudes in people working with animals and by taking the welfare of those people into account.

- Some aspects of animal treatment are improving and others are getting worse. Attention should be directed to the latter – such as methods of animal production which are still becoming more intensive – and to aspects where the impact on animals is difficult to predict – such as automation.

References

1. Rollin, B. (1993) Animal production and the new social ethic for animals. In *Food Animal Well-Being 1993: Conference Proceedings and Deliberations* (ed. Purdue University Office of Agricultural Research Programs), pp. 3–13. Purdue Research Foundation, West Lafayette.
2. Appleby, M.C. & Lawrence, A.B. (1987) Food restriction as a cause of stereotypic behaviour in tethered gilts. *Animal Production,* **45,** 103–10.
3. Harrison, J. (1998) *Effect of public feeding on behaviour of mute swans in a non-breeding flock.* MSc thesis, University of Edinburgh.
4. Waran, N.K. & Henderson, J. (1998) Stable vices: what are they and can we prevent them? *Equine Practice,* **20,** 6–8.
5. Appleby, M.C., Hughes, B.O. & Elson, H.A. (1992) *Poultry Production Systems: Behaviour, Management and Welfare.* CAB International, Wallingford, UK.
6. BVAAWF/FRAME/RSPCA/UFAW Joint Working Group on Refinements (1993) Refinements in rabbit husbandry. *Laboratory Animals,* **27,** 301–29.
7. Ames, A. (1993) *The Behaviour of Captive Polar Bears.* Universities Federation for Animal Welfare, Potters Bar, UK.
8. Professor Peter Sandøe, Chair, Danish Ethical Council for Animals, personal communication.
9. Kyriazakis, I. & Savory, C.J. (1997) Hunger and thirst. In *Animal Welfare* (eds M.C. Appleby & B.O. Hughes), pp. 49–62. CAB International, Wallingford, UK.
10. Waran, N.K. & Cuddeford, D. (1995) Effects of loading and transport on the heart rate and behaviour of horses. *Applied Animal Behaviour Science,* **43,** 71–81.
11. Waran, N.K., Robertson, V., Cuddeford, D., Kokoszko, A. & Marlin, D.J. (1996) Effects of transporting horses facing either forwards or backwards on their behaviour and heart rate. *Veterinary Record,* **139,** 7–11.
12. Gentle, M.J. (1986) Beak trimming in poultry. *World's Poultry Science Journal,* **42,** 268–275.

13. FAWC (1997) *Report on the Welfare of Laying Hens.* Farm Animal Welfare Council, Tolworth, UK.
14. Hughes, B.O. & Gentle, M.J. (1995) Beak trimming of poultry: its implications for welfare. *World's Poultry Science Journal*, **51**, 51–61.
15. Muir, W.M. (1996) Group selection for adaptation to multi-bird cages: selection program and direct responses. *Poultry Science*, **75**, 447–58.
16. Kent, J.E., Molony, V. & Robertson, I.S. (1995) Comparison of the Burdizzo and rubber ring methods of castrating and tail-docking lambs. *Veterinary Record*, **136**, 192–6.
17. Government Statistical Service (1998) *Home Office Statistics of Scientific Procedures on Living Animals in Great Britain, 1997.* Her Majesty's Stationery Office, London.
18. Mukerjee, M. (1997) Trends in animal research. *Scientific American*, February, 70–7.
19. John Finch, Chief Veterinary Officer, Inveresk Research International Ltd, personal communication.
20. Sharpe, R. (1988) *The Cruel Deception: The Use of Animals in Medical Research.* Thorsons, Wellingborough, UK.
21. RSPCA (1998) *Animals in Scientific Research – the Statistics.* RSPCA, Horsham, UK.
22. Banner Committee (1995) *Report of the Committee to Consider the Ethical Implications of Emerging Technologies in the Breeding of Farm Animals.* Her Majesty's Stationery Office, London.
23. Davis, H. and Perusse, R. (1988) Human-based social interaction can reward a rat's behaviour. *Animal Learning and Behavior*, **16**, 89–92.
24. Hemsworth, P.H., Barnett, J.L. & Coleman, G.J. (1993) The human–animal relationship in agriculture and its consequences for the animal. *Animal Welfare*, **2**, 33–51.
25. Hemsworth, P.H., Coleman, G.J. & Barnett, J.L. (1994) Improving the attitude and behaviour of stockpersons towards pigs and the consequences on the behaviour and reproductive performance of commercial pigs. *Applied Animal Behaviour Science*, **39**, 349–62.
26. Dr Alistair Lawrence, Scottish Agricultural College, Edinburgh, personal communication.
27. Bateson, P.P.G. (1997) *The Behavioural and Physiological Effects of Culling Red Deer.* Report to the Council of the National Trust.
28. Ipema, A.H., Lippus, A.C., Metz, J.H.M. & Rossing, W. (eds) (1992) *Prospects for Automatic Milking.* Pudoc Scientific Publications, Wageningen, The Netherlands.
29. Wathes, C.M. (1993) Animals in man's environment: a question of interest. In *Livestock Environment IV: Fourth International Symposium* (eds E. Collins & C. Boon), pp. 1255–66. American Society of Agricultural Engineers, St Joseph, Michigan.

Chapter 8
Buying power: Individual action

Taking the narrow way

Do you always watch the television rather than going to the cinema? Do you eat simply at home rather than going to a restaurant? Do you patch your old clothes rather than buying new ones? Some people have to do all these things, because they don't have enough money to do otherwise. Most of us, though, have room to manoeuvre in how we use our time and money. Many of our decisions are casual: few people have a policy on how much they will spend on cinema tickets each month. Others are more serious: deciding to sell the car and use public transport would take rather more thought.

The same sorts of decisions are involved in doing more for animal welfare. There are minor decisions: Shall I buy free range eggs today? There are major ones: Shall I buy a dog or a drum-kit? One vital point to note is that while the major decisions are difficult (Shall I become a vegetarian?) we mustn't let this inhibit us from taking the minor decisions. The effects of minor decisions add up. Half a loaf is better than no bread. Indeed, sometimes the half loaf of compromise is the best that can be achieved in the real world – as the discussion of animal housing established in Chapter 6.

The decisions and actions we take as individuals are important, both for our own integrity and for their effects, direct and indirect. While some of those decisions and actions need time or money, some just require a change of attitude.

This book might have been called 'What should be done about animal welfare?' But that sounds as if whatever should be done, should be done by someone else. On the contrary, we must all do something, as Chapter 1 made clear: those with special respon-

149

sibility (farmers, scientists, politicians), those with special interest (certain philosophers, welfare activists), and the general public.

In fact everyone is to some degree in the first category, with special responsibility, because we all interact with animals. Furthermore, we can move between categories: some people do make a major decision of this sort. The founders of the campaigning organization Compassion in World Farming (CIWF), Peter and Anna Roberts, were dairy and poultry farmers until they decided they didn't like the business that gave them their living.[1] And every member of CIWF or the RSPCA, including those most active, has at some stage made the decision to join those societies.

Groups may take actions, but so may people acting on their own. The question most often raised about individual action in relation to animal welfare is, to be or not to be a vegetarian.

We are what we eat

There are many arguments for and against vegetarianism that have nothing to do with animal welfare. For example, philosopher John Hill, in a book called *The Case for Vegetarianism*, presents not only 'the argument from the rights and interests of animals' but also:

> The argument from personal health,
> The argument from global ecology and
> The argument from world hunger.[2]

Conversely, vegetarianism is inconsistent with pressures for organic farming, because animals can feed on ground and plants that cannot be used for human food production, and their dung can be used to return nutrients to the soil – although not as many animals are needed for this as we keep currently.

But this is not the place to explore such arguments. Rather, we must ask here whether vegetarianism will reduce the suffering of food animals. Chapter 4 concluded that it will not, at least not directly. It will reduce the numbers of animals kept for food, but it will not itself improve the conditions in which the remainder are kept. However, it is important to remember that many people concerned about animal welfare are at least sympathetic to animal rights and dislike the idea of killing animals, so it is difficult to dissociate these approaches.

However, we have fallen into what Hill calls 'the fallacy of black and white thinking'. He defends a vegetarian who swats a fly or wears leather shoes from the charge of inconsistency or hypocrisy on the grounds that:

Complete consistency is not always possible in the real world. What is important is that she is making a real effort to live by her beliefs. In short, she may not always be consistent, but is the only other alternative to absolute consistency to make no attempt at all? Is it not better to make even modest strides in the direction to which one aspires, even if one cannot always reach one's aspiration, than to make no attempt at all?

Similarly, decisions about eating meat do not have to be all-or-nothing. We can eat less meat. We can choose meat from animals kept in extensive conditions rather than those reared intensively – for example, beef or lamb rather than pork or chicken. We can buy from organic farms rather than big companies – because organic specifications include welfare standards. We can look for products from special schemes such as the RSPCA's Freedom Foods.[3] We can favour food from wild animals, caught and killed as humanely as possible, rather than farm stock. It is also arguable that we should eat more fish – particularly farmed fish – rather than mammals and birds, on the grounds that their welfare is more easily provided for (Chapter 3).

The point is that suffering of food animals should be reduced. Until or unless that happens generally we should use our time and money to support such a change. It is interesting to note that becoming a vegetarian saves money, although it may take more time to find, prepare and cook alternatives to meat. On the other hand, finding and buying meat from animals with reasonable welfare takes both time and money. It seems a reasonable compromise to eat less meat but then to make sure that it has come from animals treated as humanely as possible. This is likely to cost about the same as a higher intake of cheaper meat. In fact, it would seem generally appropriate for us to keep fewer farm animals, to keep them better and to pay more for their meat.

In the passage quoted in Chapter 4, Singer says that vegetarianism is a boycott of factory farming. Well yes, but it is also a boycott of organic farmers and the like. It seems to suggest that all farming should be humane before we can eat a single animal.

Clearly that is an unworkable argument, because someone has to buy the more humanely reared animals to provide the incentive for that sector to expand.

Favouring extensively reared over intensively reared meat may not have the clarion-call slogan value of being able to say 'I'm a vegetarian.' However, it may actually be more persuasive, if backed up with full arguments. It is, of course, important to talk about these matters to others who may be persuaded.

Furthermore, such an approach does make a direct difference too. This is most obvious so far in relation to eggs rather than meat.

People buying free range eggs and eggs from other systems that do not use cages, for reasons that include the welfare of the hens, have caused the production of such eggs in northern Europe to increase considerably over the last 20 years. There is room for confusion here, because most people are not fully familiar with the labels used on eggs (Box 8.1). However, in the UK, attitudes among customers on this matter, combined with pressure from groups such as Compassion in World Farming, have led several major supermarket chains to label 'Eggs from Caged Hens' as such. Furthermore, Safeway supermarkets have been offering barn eggs at the same price as cage eggs, which has resulted in another large increase in their sales.

It has to be said that the welfare advantages of such systems are not clear: cages have disadvantages (Fig. 8.1), but so do other systems (Chapter 6). Nevertheless, at least these people are providing poultry farmers with the opportunity and the incentive to change their practices.

It is also striking that more people say they think battery cages should be banned than actually buy eggs from other systems.[4] That is understandable: presumably they would accept a change in legislation that increased everyone's grocery bill, not just their own, without too much complaint. However, it would be good if they, too, could put their money where their mouth is.

Supermarkets are sensitive to the concerns of their customers. To give another example, the concerns of British shoppers are currently resulting in improvements to the welfare of Danish pigs. On British pig farms, tethers and stalls for pregnant sows are now banned. On Danish farms they are not yet banned, but these farms export a huge amount of pork and bacon to the UK. The British supermarkets are confident that their customers would not like to buy meat imported from farms with lower

---

Box 8.1   European rules on egg labels

European legislation on marketing has had more impact than direct legislation on housing on how hens are kept. For example, there is no legal limit on stocking density of housed hens, but to sell 'deep litter eggs', you must not exceed the stated figure. Only the following categories are permitted:

Free range	Must have access to ground mainly covered with vegetation, with maximum of 1000 hens per hectare
Semi-intensive	As free range, but with up to 4000 hens per hectare
Deep litter	In a house with at least a third of the floor covered with litter, and maximum of 7 hens per square metre. This category is popular in Germany and The Netherlands where it is translated as 'scratching eggs'
Perchery or barn	In a house with perches that allow birds to use different levels, so up to 25 hens per square metre are allowed

Most other eggs, for example those labelled 'Farm fresh', come from cages. Occasionally if there are more barn eggs, say, than can be sold by name, they will be sold unlabelled. However, supermarkets are increasingly labelling 'Eggs from Caged Hens'.

---

standards than our own, so they are requiring the Danes to make the same changes.

Some people reading this book will be vegetarian, for a variety of reasons. If your main concern is animal welfare, you may feel that it would never be appropriate to eat an animal unless it had genuinely had 'a good life and a gentle death'. Ironically, if that is true, with the animal being treated carefully as an individual, then killing that animal for food may actually seem more objectionable rather than less. But if you are not vegetarian, you can go part of the way down this road and still have an impact: perhaps you will feel, for example, that you can choose Freedom Food or equivalent products sometimes, but not every time. That will

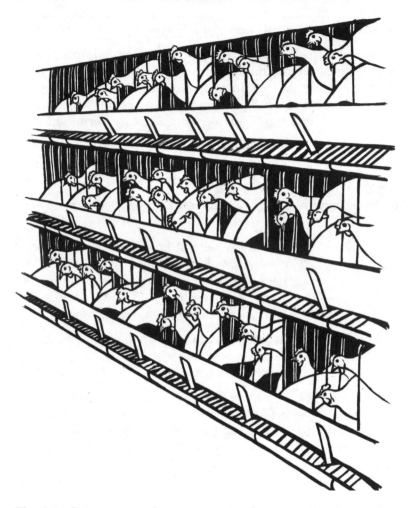

Fig. 8.1 Battery cages have many disadvantages for the welfare of hens, and buying eggs from other systems encourages change in the industry even though such systems also have disadvantages.

contribute. The effects of minor decisions add up. As the RSPCA puts it:

> If you buy Freedom Food labelled products, more shops will sell them, more farmers will produce them and more farm animals will benefit. Freedom Food gives *you* the chance to vote with your purse.[3]

You pays your money

There is a myth perpetuated by large companies that 'the public wants cheaper products', which suggests that people want cheapness at the expense of all other considerations and that cutting prices is an end that justifies all possible means. The truth, of course, is that selling their products cheaply is their major weapon in fighting other large companies in the so-called free market.

If there are two products side-by-side on the supermarket shelf with no discernible difference except in their price, naturally you tend to buy the cheaper. But if you find that it is poorer quality and if you are not on the poverty line, next time you will balance quality against price. The price difference may have other correlates too: it may be that the cheaper product is produced by a large company that can cut its margins finer than a smaller company. Many of these factors interact; for example, animal welfare will often be better on small farms than on large ones, because a farmer with 50 pigs can look after them better – can give them more space, among other things – than one with 500.

It is difficult to juggle ethical arguments while shopping, especially as shoppers concerned about animal welfare are also likely to be concerned about other ethical issues raised by their purchases, such as the conditions of workers producing the goods in developing countries. Most of us would prefer someone else to look after such matters before the goods reach the shops – to ensure, for example, that the food on sale is safe to eat and produced under humane conditions giving a reasonable living to its producers. Such actions by 'someone else' will be discussed in Chapter 9. But meanwhile, don't give up. Read the labels on the products you buy, and read them carefully: we can all be fooled at times by subtle marketing terms (do you always notice the difference between 'recycled' and 'recyclable'?). The effects of minor decisions add up. Drug and cosmetic companies that are 'Against animal testing' are making a difference, slowly but surely.

The same applies to other decisions that you make about spending your money. Money talks, and it talks louder if you spend it in the most productive ways than if you withhold it. This is not to say that decisions are easy. For example, people who disapprove of zoos and therefore don't visit them are actually foregoing their influence on how those zoos behave – in the same way that vegetarians are not directly helping the welfare of farm animals. Zoos with more money can look after their animals better. Now if the cause of the disapproval is the very act of keeping animals in captivity, then the conditions for those animals are a minor issue (although then the money might be better donated to a conservation charity). But if the problem is how animals are kept, then it might be better to keep visiting a zoo and to keep commenting on its poor enclosures, or perhaps to visit the better zoos and wildlife parks rather than the worse ones. After all, as we said in Chapter 6, most zoos have improved considerably over recent years, largely in response to public opinion. They survive on their entrance money, yet their role in education – particularly in encouraging children to have a positive attitude to animals – continues to be vital.

Similar arguments apply to circuses. Circuses are not intrinsically cruel, despite occasional unacceptable acts of cruelty such as the recent case in which a leading member of a well-known UK circus was filmed beating a tiger with an iron bar. Marthe Kiley-Worthington surveyed a number of circuses and reports that most training of animals is done gently and positively rather than by dominating and ill-treating them, which makes sense because positive training is easier and more effective. Furthermore, she believes that circuses also have an educational role:

> ... to put across the idea of the animal as an intelligent, able and beautiful sentient individual; perhaps more intelligent, able and beautiful than we had previously supposed.[5]

This means that acts should show the natural abilities of animals rather than, for example, dressing them up in silly clothes. In addition, she encourages circuses to allow people to see the animals being trained, and to visit them in their menagerie after the show, which all adds to the pressure for better treatment of the animals. She concludes:

> On balance, I do not think that the animals' best interests are necessarily served by money and activities diverted to try and ban circuses or zoos either locally or nationally. What is much more important is to continue to encourage the zoos and circuses to improve their animal welfare, and to back some inspection to ensure certain criteria are met in the animal keeping and housing.

You pays your money and you takes your choice, as the old phrase has it. Money talks, and you can help it to say the right things.

Hands on

We also interact directly with animals ourselves – with pets, pests and wildlife – and the message here is similar again: Think about it. How does what you do affect the animals concerned?

Hunting is a case in point. Few readers of this book will be active in hunting, but it is not self-evident that hunting is incompatible with welfare: different types of hunting differ in their effects on welfare. Shooting a deer, in a population that is too large and has to be controlled, causes few welfare problems if skilfully done. Furthermore, reduction of a population surplus can potentially be done just as well by a paying client as by a paid stalker. On the other hand, pheasant shooting (Fig. 8.2) is less acceptable.[6] Birds are reared and released specially for shooting, and welfare problems occur during both these processes. There can be up to 80% mortality in the 4 weeks after release, because the birds are not fitted for life in the wild. Then the shooting itself causes suffering, because a proportion of birds are injured rather than killed. Lastly, chasing a deer or a fox with dogs is certainly harmful.[7]

Interactions with other wildlife also require thought. We have already talked about the people who feed the ducks in good weather, but not on the cold days when they need food the most (Chapter 7). If you feed the birds in your garden so regularly that they come to rely on you, what happens if you go away for a week's skiing in midwinter? Is bread the best food for birds in the breeding season?

But for most people the biggest question that directly affects animals is to keep or not to keep a pet? The decision should not be a casual one. Find out about the animal and its needs. Read books such as the one produced by the Waltham Centre for Pet Nutrition, on *Benefits and Responsibilities of Pet Ownership*.[8] Talk to others about the problems – the problems both for you and for the animal. Plan how you can avoid leaving the pet alone for long periods, particularly highly social animals such as dogs and horses. If there are likely to be major problems, don't get a pet. Remember that this will be a two-sided relationship. When we are considering whether to have a child we have to consider the

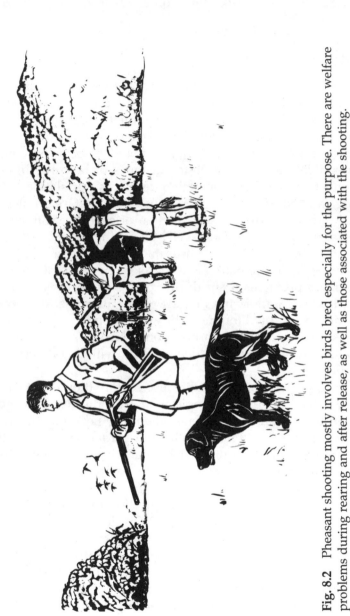

Fig. 8.2 Pheasant shooting mostly involves birds bred especially for the purpose. There are welfare problems during rearing and after release, as well as those associated with the shooting.

child's needs, not just our own, and the same is true with pets. Looking after a pet properly takes a lot of work, and with larger pets a lot of money too.

Given due thought and commitment, a decision to keep a pet seems reasonable. A pet can have what certainly seems to be a happy life. Remember too, though, that in due course you will probably also have to take responsibility for her death. It is not fair to keep her alive for your benefit once it is no benefit to her to continue living.

It is a two-sided relationship: people gain considerable pleasure from pets, and pets may also be beneficial to health. For example, old people show many signs of reduced stress if they own a dog or a cat,[9] and pets may also have positive influences on the development of children.[10] Furthermore, educational value must also be important. It is useful for children to learn that parental disapproval will follow if they tease the cat, as well as if they are mean to each other. Although it is not clear where the cause and effect lie, children who have pets (Fig. 8.3) are more likely as adults to have positive attitudes to animals.[11]

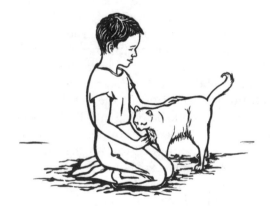

Fig. 8.3 A relationship with a pet can help a child to develop a positive attitude towards animals, including responsibility for their care.

Our duty to animals can be illustrated by this summary of our responsibilities to dogs:

> The quality of the dog's life is the total responsibility of the owner ... There are a number of basic obligations which all owners should fulfil.
> The dog is a social animal and the owner needs to spend

several hours per day interacting with it. In addition, dogs need to be stimulated mentally, not only through training of basic commands but also through 'games' designed to employ their cognitive abilities. Dogs need to be exercised every day ... Owners are also responsible for the physical health requirements of their dogs ... Dog ownership, like the rearing of children, requires dedication, understanding, time and effort, and the responsibilities last a lifetime.[12]

A single step

The longest journey begins with a single step, and in the case of animal welfare one useful step is joining an animal welfare charity. It is worth remembering here that minor decisions are worth taking even if major decisions in the background are daunting or off-putting: it is worth taking the single step even if you don't know whether you want to make the whole journey. Many people say that they don't join charitable societies because they wouldn't have the time or commitment to participate in all the activities. That is a mistake. It is better to join the society, so that it can use your subscription fee and quote its increased membership, than not to join it. Whether you contribute to the activities is a separate decision that can be taken later.

Some people also object to the idea of animal charities, or to the idea of making donations to them, on the grounds that there is so much human suffering in the world. Certainly the occasional story of someone leaving all their millions to a dogs' home does seem to indicate rather antisocial, misanthropic character. However, support for animal welfare and human welfare are not mutually exclusive. Few would object to a Last Will and Testament that left money to both a famine-relief agency and an animal welfare fund. Most of us could do more for charity. The argument here is that we should increase our charitable giving or effort for animals, not that we should reduce that for humans.

What other single steps can you make? Well, some charities are particularly strong on recommending involvement by their members. Compassion in World Farming, for example, has suggestions for action in every issue of their magazine *Agscene*, such as writing letters to politicians and quizzing your milk supplier about the welfare of the cows from which the milk comes. There are books specializing in just this in most bookshops. You are unlikely to agree with all the opinions of any one society, or with all the suggestions of any one such book, but you will find some contribution you can make.

Perhaps most importantly, educate both yourself and your children – or help to educate any children with whom you have any influence. It is depressing to see children throwing stones at pigeons while their parents sit by without interfering. It is good to see families at the zoo and to hear them talking about conservation, animal care and the things that really matter to animals. Today's children are tomorrow's users, abusers or protectors of animals.

Taking the bull by the horns

Having looked at some of the responsible decisions and actions to be taken, we must also give some consideration to irresponsible actions and those of dubious responsibility. It is ironic, given that the issue of animal protection is about humane behaviour and ethical standards, that the banners of animal rights and animal liberation have often been associated with extremism and lawbreaking. To give a recent example, in August 1998 members of the Animal Liberation Front released 6000 mink from a fur farm in the south of England, smashing cages and cutting wire.[13] The case caused a furore among landowners and wildlife specialists, with many of the released animals either being run over or shot by local farmers. Those that survived will have a major impact on the ecosystem: they soon started killing not only prey species but even owls at a local owl sanctuary. Escaped mink have previously had serious effects on wildlife throughout the UK, including contributing to the decline of wild otters by competing for their food resources. The action was condemned by the RSPCA and by other groups such as Respect for Animals, who pointed out that the British government is already committed to phasing out fur farming in the UK.

A representative of the ALF defended the action:

> I know many of them are going to die, but at least they will have had a taste of freedom. If they had stayed in the fur farm, every one of them would have been killed. And the ones who survive will hopefully live their lives out in a natural environment.[13]

At best this was a partial argument. The 'taste of freedom' would have been frightening rather than exhilarating, and any benefits to those that survive will be offset by problems for other species.

It is undeniable that such actions have achieved publicity for the cause of animal protection. This case reminded the public that fur farming still existed in Britain and probably increased the pressure on the government to stand by its commitment to ending it. Yet extremism is also counterproductive. Thus many moderate people who feel strongly about animals join moderate organizations such as the RSPCA, but more would probably do so if they weren't repelled from the whole issue by the extremists.

Furthermore, choosing to break those laws with which you disagree is by definition anarchy. After all, other people have other priorities. Rather, we should seek to change the law.

That said, there is a long tradition of argument that it is sometimes appropriate to break laws which appear to be unjust, if there seems to be no other way of presenting a serious challenge to The System. This argument was made most famously by Henry Thoreau, who wrote *On the Duty of Civil Disobedience* in the 1850s.[14] However, there are two key points to be made here. People who follow this route must firstly be sure that they really have no alternative – which certainly does not apply to an act of criminal damage on a fur farm that is anyway condemned to closure. Secondly, they must be prepared to answer for their actions within the rest of the legal system.

An event that seems to fulfil all reasonable criteria for such civil disobedience occurred in Australia in October 1995. Members of a group called Animal Liberation entered a battery farm at night, without causing any damage. They found a number of sick and dead birds in the cages, which they took to a vet. Then they called the police and the media and allowed themselves to be arrested. They were prosecuted for trespass but pleaded 'reasonable excuse' on grounds that were later summarized by the magistrate:

> Despite the more traditional lobbying tactics they had employed for many years, what they believed to be the barbaric practice of extracting eggs from hens in circumstances amounting to cruelty continued. Their argument is that, in these circumstances, some mildly unlawful attention-grabbing behaviour is excusable.[15]

He accepted their plea, commenting that the group had not impeded the work of the farm: they had, indeed, helped in identifying birds needing removal, culling or treatment. Furthermore, he accepted their argument that battery cages were cruel, conforming to some aspects of the law but contravening others:

> Portia argued successfully, and with popular acclaim, that Shylock could extract his pound of flesh provided that it caused no harm and provided that no blood was spilt. It is not a fanciful argument to say that you may only raise hens in a battery of cages provided that, in so doing, no harm was caused, the hens were given adequate exercise, allowed to stretch, nest, ruffle, etc.[16]

The case is still going through the appeal process, but it has had an additional effect of causing discussion at all levels in the courts about the accusations of cruelty as well as those of trespass.

A final point to make about protest action, then, is that communication is vital. Peter Singer makes this point in a review of a book called *The Art of Moral Protest:*

> While painting 'the enemy' in an entirely negative light may help to boost morale within the movement, it often means that the movement loses touch with reality and misses opportunities to communicate with those who are in a position to make a difference. In the animal movement, for instance, Henry Spira has been uniquely effective in eliminating or reducing the abuse of animals precisely because, instead of demonising research scientists at corporations like Revlon, Avon and Proctor & Gamble, he has assumed that they are ordinary people, who will be prepared to find a way to reduce animal suffering if they can find a way of doing it without causing serious damage to the interests of the organisation for which they work.[16]

Individual communications and actions add up to have an effect. Furthermore, individual opinions, and participation in lobbying, add up to influence the wider ways in which society treats animals. Those ways are the subject of the next chapter.

Conclusions

- Exercising our individual responsibility for animal welfare may involve major decisions, but if those are difficult we should not be put off taking minor decisions. Effects of minor decisions add up. This is true in relation to how we use our money, whether shopping or visiting zoos or joining welfare societies. It is also true with regard to actions that increase awareness of animal welfare issues.

- Buying meat and other animal products from producers with high welfare standards does more to improve the welfare of farm animals than does vegetarianism. The attitudes and buying patterns of customers influence the actions of super-markets in setting such standards, and are critical to the success of quality assurance schemes such as the RSPCA's Freedom Foods.

- Direct involvement with animals, for example by keeping pets, can benefit the animals and is also important in learning and exercising responsible animal care.

- Moderate welfare organizations say that actions by extremists slow down progress on animal welfare rather than promoting it. The main purpose of protest action should be not immediate gains but communication and publicity, changing attitudes and influencing policy makers.

References

1. D'Silva, J. (1997) Agscene Interview. *Agscene (The Quarterly Magazine of Compassion in World Farming)*, Autumn, 14–5.
2. Hill, J.L. (1996) *The Case for Vegetarianism: Philosophy for a Small Planet*. Rowman & Littlefield, Maryland.
3. RSPCA (undated) *Freedom Food leaflet*. Freedom Foods Ltd, West Sussex, UK.
4. Bennett, R. (1997) Consumer perception and poultry welfare. In *Proceedings of the 5th European Symposium on Poultry Welfare* (eds P. Koene & H.J. Blokhuis), pp. 179–81.
5. Kiley-Worthington, M. (1990) *Animals in Circuses and Zoos: Chiron's World?* Little Eco-Farms, Basildon, UK.
6. Faure, J.M., Melin, J.M. & Mantovani, C. (1993) Welfare of guinea fowl and game birds. In *Proceedings of the 4th European Symposium on Poultry Welfare* (eds C.J. Savory & B.O. Hughes), pp. 148–57. Universities Federation for Animal Welfare, Potters Bar, UK.
7. Bateson, P.P.G. (1997) *The Behavioural and Physiological Effects of Culling Red Deer*. Report to the Council of the National Trust.

8. Robinson, I. (ed.) (1995) *The Waltham Book of Human–Animal Interaction: Benefits and Responsibilities of Pet Ownership.* Pergamon, Oxford.
9. Hart, L.A. (1995) The role of pets in enhancing human well-being: effects for older people. In *The Waltham Book of Human–Animal Interaction: Benefits and Responsibilities of Pet Ownership* (ed. I. Robinson), pp. 19–31. Pergamon, Oxford.
10. Endenburg, N. & Baarda, B. (1995) The role of pets in enhancing human well-being: effects on child development. In *The Waltham Book of Human-Animal Interaction: Benefits and Responsibilities of Pet Ownership* (ed. I. Robinson), pp. 7–17. Pergamon, Oxford.
11. Paul, E.S. & Serpell, J.A. (1993) Pet ownership in childhood: its influence on attitudes towards animals. *Applied Animal Behaviour Science,* **35**, 296.
12. McBride, A. (1995) The human-dog relationship. In *The Waltham Book of Human–Animal Interaction: Benefits and Responsibilities of Pet Ownership* (ed. I. Robinson), pp. 99–112. Pergamon, Oxford.
13. Hall, S. (1998) Farmers reach for their guns as mink run wild in New Forest. *Guardian Weekly,* 11th August.
14. Thoreau, H.D. (re-issued 1986) *Walden, or, Life in the Woods, and On the duty of Civil Disobedience.* Collier, New York.
15. Ward, M. (1997) *Reasons for Decision of Magistrate Ward Delivered on the 18th Day of February 1997.* Magistrates Court, Canberra.
16. Singer, P. (1998) The poet and the engineer (review of *The Art of Moral Protest,* by J. Jasper (1998, University of Chicago Press)). *The Times Higher Education Supplement,* 7th August, p. 23.

Chapter 9
Votes and lobbies: Action by society

Seeing the wood for the trees

So you keep a dog, and you treat it well. You feed the birds in your back garden. But how should the nation (to quote Gandhi again), or the League of Nations, treat its dogs and its birds? How should society improve its treatment of animals? If you are going to write letters, join protests and lobbies, use your vote wisely, what should you be asking for?

One way of answering these questions is similar to that for individual actions. There are both minor and major issues involved, both specific and general approaches.

It is sometimes said that ethical decisions on animal use should be made on a case-by-case basis, making a judgement on the specific features of each case. There are circumstances in which this is true. It is difficult to imagine society banning all experiments on animals (and even more difficult nowadays, thank goodness, to imagine it permitting all experiments) so it needs a mechanism to consider individual proposals. Furthermore, specific questions focus the attention: Was it right to clone Dolly the sheep? Should battery cages be banned?

However, answers to such questions are not easy. 'Every complex question has a simple answer,' as someone has said: 'simple and wrong'. Most specific changes to how we treat animals would have knock-on effects (just as they do in animal housing, as discussed in Chapter 6). This is illustrated very clearly by the issue of transport of farm animals (Fig. 9.1). This hit the British headlines in 1994 when it became widely known that calves were being exported to other countries, for rearing in veal crates that would be illegal in the UK. Large public protests started at ferry ports,

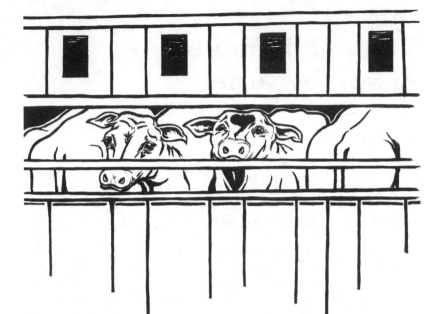

Fig. 9.1 Transport of farm animals is controversial, and rightly so. All the Five Freedoms (Box 2.4) are compromised: animals are likely to be hungry, thirsty, uncomfortable and distressed; they are restricted in behaviour and are often injured.

and the focus soon broadened to include export of live animals for slaughter.

The pressure group Compassion in World Farming was closely involved in these protests, and used journalistic licence in simplifying the picture:

> The culprits: Britain's sheep farmers who – driven by greed – are willing to see their animals hauled huge distances in overcrowded trucks only all too often to be brutally slaughtered in southern Europe. When the trade resumed at the beginning of July [1996] sheep prices in Britain were 18% higher than a year ago. Surely an 18% rise should be enough for anyone. Do sheep farmers really have to subject their animals to the miseries of live export just to squeeze a couple of extra percentage points out of them?[1]

It is in fact very unlikely that the British farmers could have sold all their stock in Britain, at any price. Furthermore, it is not just the farmers who decide where their animals go: there are several independent operators involved, including markets, hauliers and abattoirs. There are many other complications. If dairy farmers could not sell their excess calves to the highest bidder – or to any bidder at all – they would have to be slaughtered at birth, and the economics of dairying would become even more precarious. If animals had to be slaughtered near to home, there would have to be more slaughterhouses, equipped to deal with occasional large numbers of animals but able financially to cope with frequent dearth of supply.

The *principle* is right: it would be better to slaughter animals as close to their farms as possible and transport them as carcases rather than alive. But the idea that we can achieve this at a stroke is wrong.

There are specific changes that can be made, and in addition publicity about specific issues is useful for setting the mood against which decisions are made. The protests about transport probably had some effect on the subsequent decision by the EU to improve the conditions in which animals are transported (although the improvement was minor). Single issue campaigns do have the virtue of achieving more impact, more headlines, than more complex campaigns. By all means write to your MP asking for fox hunting to be banned.

But what are needed even more are broader decisions on a society-wide basis that would affect not just one issue but many related issues. It may well be, for example, that we should accept higher prices for meat, or that increased priority should be given to preventative health care – which should reduce the use of laboratory animals in developing medicines. There is no contradiction here with the argument in Chapter 2 that scientists need to concentrate on specific problems rather than overall views. In solving those problems at the level of society we need to take a broad view. We need to make sure we can see the wood as well as the trees.

Broader still

Furthermore, our own wood is only part of a larger forest. We can't ignore what happens outside our own country – particularly because international trade is continually increasing and, as mentioned in Chapter 1, attitudes to welfare differ between countries.

People in countries where concern for welfare is high must be careful when commenting on others with different priorities. For example, Alan Herscovici has written a powerful reply to those who criticize Canadian native people for trapping animals. If trapping were stopped, it would end a lifestyle that has been traditional for generations, and the response of the people involved is often forthright:

> The Inuit say that the philosophy of animal rights is merely the latest outburst of the cultural and economic imperialism they've come to expect from Europe and the South.[2]

Even more persuasively, countries that have difficulty feeding their people understandably put more emphasis on food availability than on animal welfare. Of course the situation is rarely black-and-white. Herscovici points out that:

> Bringing aboriginal trappers off their hunting territories is a crucial step towards 'clearing the land' for pipelines, power dams and other high-tech frontier 'development' projects, and all the disruption of wildlife habitat that they bring with them. For this reason, many wildlife biologists question whether the demands of the animal rights groups are even really in the interests of wildlife.[2]

Similarly, priorities other than animal welfare may sometimes influence welfare positively. Norway has legislation to limit farm size, because it regards rural employment as important, and this limitation probably has some benefits for welfare. France puts emphasis on food quality, which also has some positive effects: free-range, slower-growing broiler chickens are common.

The best strategy must be to tread softly among other people's sensibilities. There is always room for improvement. Thus, while it may be difficult or inappropriate to ban trapping of animals for fur, there has been extensive research on development of traps that are more humane than the old-fashioned gin traps.[3]

Indeed, there is considerable room for improvement on the basis of enlightened self-interest. The peasant farmer may well be short of food for himself and his family. He can still learn that he will get more work from his donkey if he cajoles her rather than beating her (Fig. 9.2).

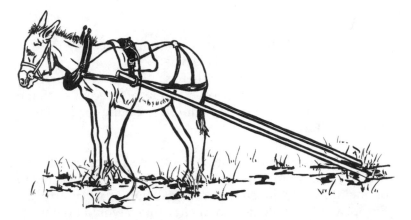

Fig. 9.2 Subsistence farmers can often benefit from improving the welfare of their animals. This donkey will work better if looked after than if maltreated.

An important paper promoting this approach has been published by Cheryl McCrindle, a South African vet. She presents what she calls an African perspective:

> This paper addresses the possibility of a paradigm shift which would result in animal welfare succeeding in its aims through making it people-centred rather than animal-centred. It looks, therefore, at the benefits that accrue to people when the well-being of animals is improved as well as the benefits that accrue to animals when the well-being of people is improved ... Sometimes it is as simple as a veterinarian supplying information on a supplementary lick or feed which results in better milk production and higher fertility of the cows. The subsistence level farming family improve their intake of butterfat and milk protein and may also earn money by selling milk to their neighbours. Because the cows are better fed they do not starve slowly to death in the dry season or suffer from disease.[4]

Such an approach, and others that promote animal welfare world-wide while being sensitive to local needs and priorities, can be furthered by governments and by welfare societies in their international communications and negotiations.

Points of law

As soon as governments come into the picture, obviously the main action to be considered is legislation.

Some animal users consider there is already too much legislation about animal welfare. For example, at a recent conference on farm animal welfare Andrew Jorêt, speaking for the UK egg industry, said that:

> Legislation is a 'blunt tool' and can be unnecessarily over-prescriptive. More importantly, it prevents progress. Because of the difficulty in changing legislation, particularly on a European basis, new developments which would give welfare benefits have little chance of ever being adopted. A preferred route to legislation is the development and use of Codes of Practice. There are two very good schemes available to egg producers – The RSPCA Freedom Food scheme for non-cage birds and the British Egg Industry Council's Lion scheme for all types of production. To be effective, Codes of Practice have to be understood by consumers … Animal welfare is, and should be, a consumer choice issue, not the producer choice issue it has often been presented as.[5]

These comments raise at least three major issues. Firstly, commercial users of animals – whether zoos or laboratories or farms – have rarely introduced 'new developments which would give welfare benefits' unless these were profitable or convenient. Nor could they be expected to do so. So the blunt tool of legislation is sometimes necessary.

Secondly, it is true that legislation is not the only route. Codes of Practice can be helpful, including voluntary codes such as the two mentioned, but again, voluntary standards will only go so far. It is ironic that these two codes are indeed optional, so they are exactly the sort of producer choice that the speaker denied was important. There is, however, a third code that applies to UK poultry producers: the Ministry of Agriculture's *Code of Recommendation for the Welfare of Domestic Fowls*.[6] This outlines standards such as stocking densities, and it does so in the form of recommendations, not regulations. But there is an important difference from the other two codes. This one is *backed* by legislation. It has the same status, in fact, as the *Highway Code*. Breaking the *Highway Code* – for example, driving on the wrong side of the road – is not itself against the law. But if you do break the *Code*, this can be used as evidence if you are accused of dangerous driving, which *is* illegal. In the same way, if a poultry farmer is accused of cruelty or neglect, the fact that he has used higher than recommended stocking densities can be used in the prosecution.

Thirdly, it may well be appropriate to describe welfare as a consumer choice issue. We are all consumers, and the consensus is that more should be done for animal welfare. The mistaken inference, though, is that any matter that involves selling should be dealt with at the point of sale. The argument goes like this: consumers who think pigs should be kept outdoors will buy outdoor-pigmeat even if it is more expensive. Most consumers in this category think that welfare of outdoor pigs is better than that of those indoors,[7] and we can set aside here the question of whether this is actually true (Chapters 2, 6). According to the argument, then, the proportion of pigs kept outdoors will come to match the proportion of people concerned about this: if that proportion increases, fair enough; if it doesn't, fair enough too: clear labelling of products is all that is necessary. The argument is wrong. Labelling is not enough.

As emphasized in Chapter 8 it is difficult to juggle ethical arguments while shopping, and many people simply don't do so. Suppose there are two products for sale, with one made in a factory that is unsafe for the workers and therefore cheaper. Many people will buy it anyway. Apart from anything else, there is a feeling – insofar as people think about it – that buying *this* product *now* will not affect the workers (or the animals) that produced it, because the production has already happened. Anyway, society decides that worker safety should be protected and legislates accordingly. It doesn't burden shoppers with day-by-day responsibility for the welfare of human food producers, nor should it do so with the welfare of the animals.

Does society want to improve animal welfare, if only a minority of shoppers buy outdoor-pigmeat? Yes it does. A majority of the remainder also wants pigs to be kept outdoors.[7] Furthermore, people who do buy such meat want *all* pigs to be kept outdoors. So, in all probability, do vegetarians.[8]

There should be more legislation to protect animal welfare, or more stringent Codes of Practice backed by legislation, or both. Countries vary in the prescriptiveness of their legislation. Some state generally that animals must not be ill-treated, but this is often difficult to apply. Others prohibit specific actions or require particular conditions. It is sometimes argued that this doesn't make very much difference overall. For instance, the EU is generally more heavy-handed with legislation than the USA, which has almost none protecting the welfare of farm animals. Some people (particularly in the USA) doubt that animals in Europe are any better off. Well, it is difficult to generalize, but there are certainly instances of better conditions for animals in Europe. As one example, the USA does not have legislation on battery cage size. As a result, most laying hens in the USA have less than $350\,cm^2$ each, compared to the statutory minimum of $450\,cm^2$ in Europe.

What should the increased legislation or strengthened Codes of Practice be about? We can summarize from the arguments of the previous chapters: better conditions for a good life and a gentle death, limitations on the harm we can do to animals and positive provisions for their welfare. As Chapter 4 said, the relationship between humans and animals is two-sided, and since we are in control it is our responsibility to look after both sides, not just our own.

Again, it's not just specific changes that matter, but general approaches too. The EU's acceptance that animals are 'sentient beings'[9] will change the way in which animal legislation is framed. For example, legislation about animal transport was previously seen just as a variant on that about transport of other property, but now it will be treated differently, in a category of its own.

The next question is: who is to legislate? For some categories of animals, particularly farm animals, that is a major problem.

Legislative supremacy

For many animals, welfare is mostly a matter for national governments, because actions within a country have relatively little effect outside. This applies to animals in laboratories, zoos, circuses, sporting centres and the countryside, as well as to pets and pests. There are some effects. If the size of laboratory cages is increased scientists may complain that their competitiveness with those in other countries is reduced, or that their results are no longer comparable with those from abroad. But these effects rarely override national sensitivities.

The situation is much more complicated for farm animals, that are kept to produce a product – primarily food. Remember that farm animals outnumber all the other categories, at least among large, land-living vertebrates. The problem is that the product can cross national boundaries, sometimes still on the hoof. More, it *must be allowed* to cross boundaries, under arrangements such as the European Union, the North American Free Trade Agreement and more recently the World Trade Organization (which arose from GATT, the General Agreement on Tariffs and Trade). These have as their main aim the free trade of goods between countries: the other name for the EU is the Common Market. So any measures improving animal welfare that mean the product has to be sold at a higher price may lead to problems of competition from other countries that do not have similar measures.

Banning sow stalls and tethers in the UK from January 1999 is likely to increase the selling price of British pigmeat and encourage imports of cheaper meat from countries without a similar ban (although this will be affected by the policies of supermarkets discussed in Chapter 8). This is often referred to as 'exporting our welfare problems'.

So do we lie down and let free trade trample over us and our animals? No, we tackle this problem at all possible levels. It doesn't help to exaggerate the problem. Andrew Jorêt, quoted above, went on to talk about EU proposals for improving welfare of battery hens:

> There is no point in legislating our own industry out of existence only to turn round and import that product from those very same systems, but operated to much lower standards than were in use at home.[5]

The phrase about 'legislating our own industry out of existence' is an overstatement. Denmark has had more stringent legislation on battery cages than the rest of Europe for years: it requires $600\,\mathrm{cm}^2$ per bird rather than $450\,\mathrm{cm}^2$. When the legislation was introduced the Danish egg industry contracted – it went from being a net exporter of eggs to a net importer – but it did not die. Similarly, Jorêt said elsewhere in his talk that there is little likelihood of many fresh eggs being imported to the EU, as they would no longer be fresh when they got here. The particular danger is that imports of processed eggs – which make up 25% of European egg production – would rise. So again, European egg production might shrink under the proposed changes, but it would not disappear. Shrinkage is not a trivial matter, but in view of the continuing overproduction of food in many parts of the developed world, the threat of shrinkage in agricultural production is not an unanswerable argument either.

There is a strong argument for at least some practices that it is appropriate to 'put our own house in order' – to proceed with legislation at a national level despite international pressures, and in Europe at EU level despite world-wide pressures. Obviously this must take account of the economic impact, and proceed in parallel with measures to ameliorate the impact. But economics must not be the sole arbiter of our actions.

Sweden is currently in the process of banning barren cages for laying hens. They are requiring producers to provide hens with nest boxes and loose material, whether they do so in enriched cages (Chapter 6) or in other systems. They are doing this despite the fact that they won't be able to prevent import of cheaper eggs from elsewhere in the EU (but see p. 118). It is my opinion, having worked for many years on this subject, that all countries should do the same. It is my opinion as a British citizen that even if other countries do not do so, the UK should follow Sweden in this matter.

We have already discussed one major factor that will reduce the impact of economics. Although we said just now that changing UK legislation on pig housing is likely to increase the price of pork and encourage imports, those imports will actually be limited by the fact that supermarkets are sensitive to the concerns of their customers on this matter (Chapter 8). The fact that marketing is not just a simple matter of the lowest possible pricing will be discussed below.

Another approach to the problem of free trade is to strive for change outside our borders as well as inside. Other countries may change their practices for various reasons, and one of them is the opportunity to increase or retain their share of our markets – as Danish pig producers are doing for UK sales. Of course European countries must strive to convince fellow-members of the EU to share their views. Of course we must strive to shape the WTO to suit our own priorities. European countries (perhaps particularly the UK) tend to talk as if the EU is an outside agency, whereas each country is an equal participant. Similarly, we are all joint architects of the WTO, and can all contribute to its future shape.

Lastly, we can find ways of circumventing free trade. For example, one mechanism for improving welfare that has received less attention than it justifies is careful use of public money. John Webster makes concrete proposals on this in relation to farm animals:

All attempts, such as those within the Council of Europe, to devise legislation to improve the welfare of the laying hen have, so far, been obsessed with the need to define minimum standards for cage design. There is, however, a much more attractive way to achieve the same objective, namely improved living standards for the laying hen. This is to devise financial incentives and penalties designed to shift the economic balance in favour of alternative systems such as a subsidy for producers who kept birds on free range with flock sizes no larger than 200 birds ... In 1993, 42% of income to farmers within the European Union came from government grants and subsidies using taxpayers' money. At present many subsidies, such as those for extensification and set-aside, are dictated almost entirely by the need to avoid overproduction. There is some emphasis on the maintenance of environmental quality and living standards for the small farmer but, at present, no example of subsidy directly designed to maintain the quality of life on the land, and this should imply quality of life for both farmers and their animals. I suggest most strongly that matters of animal welfare should be central to any discussion as to the best use of agricultural subsidy.[10]

Some such subsidies are already in place, for example for organic production with its higher welfare standards, particularly in certain countries such as Germany. If a subsidy does not reduce the selling price of the product, it will not contravene the principles of the free market. At the very least, it's worth exploring.

We have all still got a lot of exploring to do, finding ways of fulfilling our responsibilities to animals. Politicians must be explorers too.

Trade marks

Politicians make laws on our behalf for producers. They also make them for other people with commercial involvement with animals: hauliers, slaughterers and traders.

Furthermore, in some instances traders can act where governments cannot. During the controversy over export of live animals from the UK in 1994–1996 the British government was unable to interfere in the free trade between EU countries. Ferry companies could decide, however, to stop carrying animals, and most of them did so.

As we have seen, companies – perhaps particularly super-markets – have a part to play in improving animal welfare. Labelling is not enough, but it does contribute. Schemes such as the RSPCA's Freedom Food are having an increasing impact: in the UK over 3500 production companies have joined Freedom Foods since its launch in 1994 and the products are stocked by about 4000 stores.[11] It is clear that while there may be consensus among many people in many countries that animal welfare should be improved, there is no universal consensus about how much it should be improved, or at what cost. To some extent, therefore, people and countries will have to agree to differ, at least for the foreseeable future. Products associated with different levels of animal welfare will continue to coexist on our super-market shelves for now.

Supermarkets can also take decisions with broader impact than just offering customers choice, as in the example of those stocking only free range eggs or pricing barn eggs favourably (Chapter 8). Clearly these are still primarily marketing decisions. These stores are aiming their marketing at the general wishes of their regular customers (or the people who might become their regular cus-tomers), as established by buying patterns and market research. This does not just apply to food. It also applies to other products with an impact on animal welfare, such as cosmetics: the com-pany Beauty Without Cruelty captures a sector of the market and the Body Shop gives major publicity to a similar policy. These are marketing decisions, but they may also be ethically based.

The worrying aspect is that where marketing decisions are not ethically based, they may change rapidly in relation to market forces or the current perception of those forces. An example occurred in the UK in 1998. Several supermarket chains had agreed to buy pork from a list of farms which reared pigs under specified conditions, in an arrangement called the Malton con-tract.[12] When the market changed and the price of pork fell, the supermarkets withdrew from the contract unilaterally. This left the farmers, many of whom had altered their farms to meet the contract, without buyers. The same could happen with many agreements more specifically aimed at safeguarding animal welfare.

The point has been well made with regard to the related topic of fair trade – trade that is fair for the people producing products in developing countries:

> Ethical consumerism is, at its core, a reflection of public concern to create a better world. But, in the era of globalisation, ethical consumers need to look beyond the supermarket shelf – and beyond appeals for voluntary action by powerful corporations. What is needed now is a new system of world trade rules that prioritise the needs of people and the environment over the dictates of free trade.[13]

To the needs of people and the environment in that passage, we can – and we should – add the needs of animals.

It's good to talk

In all these decision-making processes, communication is vital – as was emphasized in Chapter 1. At a basic level, information about all the issues considered in this book is spreading. Not long ago most people literally did not know that 'Farm Fresh Eggs' come from battery cages, because they did not think about it, because they did not want to think about it. The level of awareness is probably increasing now, but slowly.

Apart from media interest in this area, many societies and charities are involved in the spread of information. The Humane Society of the US runs Farm Animal Awareness Week.[14] The Association for Study of Animal Behaviour, based in the UK, provides videos and other support for school teaching on animal behaviour and welfare.[15] The Universities Federation for Animal Welfare produces handbooks for the management of farm and laboratory animals,[16] among many other publications, and the Scientists Center for Animal Welfare does similar work in the USA.

This level of communication must be maintained and extended, among those with special responsibility for welfare, those with special interest, and the general public. Accessible information is important whether you want to keep cows, or horses, or iguanas.

Furthermore, this communication must be based on understanding. As just one example, there has been a lot of heated discussion in the media and elsewhere of the rights and wrongs of genetic engineering. Much of this heat has been generated by misunderstanding, but not necessarily misunderstanding of genetic engineering. Here are two of the many likely areas. First, opponents tend to say 'We don't like the idea of altering the genetic foundation of animals' biology'. Proponents reply 'But it is useful'. If that is the level of communication, never the twain shall meet, because the two arguments use fundamentally different ethical approaches. One asks whether the *action* is right or wrong, whereas the other emphasizes the *consequences* (Chapter 1).

Secondly, proponents of many types of genetic engineering, such as the production of medicines in sheep milk, argue that it doesn't cause any suffering to the animals (Chapter 5). They may, nevertheless, not persuade opponents that it is acceptable, if the opponents' view of welfare puts more emphasis on naturalness than on feelings or health – on animal natures rather than animal minds or bodies (Chapter 2).

Understanding may not generate agreement, but it is necessary if communication is to be meaningful. Communication must be mutual: it should not be conducted through a megaphone. In the last section of the book we turn to the subject of dialogue, to consider how we can ascertain the consensus which is the very basis of not only the book but the whole justification for improving animal welfare.

Consensus and accountability

Many people say that they dislike committees, and it is true that at its worst a committee can be a mechanism for wasting time rather than getting on with the job. However, at its best a committee can use its varied membership to obtain relevant information, come to a consensus (as distinct from a majority vote) and explain the basis for its decisions. Here we shall consider different sorts of committee, and whether there should be more overlap between these categories.

One of the most encouraging ideas in recent years has been the Consensus Conference. This approach was developed in Denmark, and the first such conference in the UK was held in 1994, on plant biotechnology. A committee or panel of lay people was first briefed over 3 months about the science and issues involved. They then put questions to representatives of the industry and consumer groups, environmentalists and ethicists. Finally they came up with recommendations, for example that:

There should be an internationally recognized organization which oversees multinational developments and ensures that they will not have an adverse impact on developing countries.[17]

One observer commented that:

For me, the conclusions of the panel of 16, produced through all this process of briefing and questioning, with contributions from people of all persuasions in the audience, carried far more weight than a referendum with a set of unexplained and possibly loaded questions.[17]

In Denmark, the conclusions of such conferences are used in decisions about public policy. That is not yet the case in the UK or other countries, but this practice could valuably be adopted.

Then there are committees that do actually make important recommendations and decisions. One of the problems in understanding how decisions are made is that these committees are many and varied, even within one country. In the UK some are temporary, such as the Banner Committee which considered the ethics of breeding techniques for farm animals.[18] Some are permanent and advisory, such as the Farm Animal Welfare Council. Some have more immediate effect on policy, such as the Animal Procedures Committee that advises the Home Office on the types of experiment that should be permitted. There is a committee of members of parliament on welfare and a minister with special responsibility for the subject.

What is missing, though, is comprehensiveness and consensus. The coverage of these committees is patchy. Some subjects, such as the welfare of pets, are not obviously covered at all. Others are considered within relatively narrow guidelines. It is not apparent, for example, whether any of these committees could consider the broad questions we raised above, about whether we should pay more for meat, or give more priority to preventative health care. Michael Banner and his group recommended:

That an advisory committee be created, whose remit should include a responsibility for broad ethical questions relating to current and future developments in the use of animals.[18]

Such a committee was described as 'an ethical watchdog' in the press,[19] but the recommendation was rejected by the government.

The Banner group's opinion that an ethical advisory committee on animals is necessary is endorsed by the arguments of this book and this chapter, with the slight modification that whereas Banner was primarily considering biotechnology it is clear that all issues affecting animal welfare need to be addressed in this way. This book therefore recommends that animal welfare ethical advisory committees should be established by national governments, with international communication and collaboration being expected and encouraged. In the UK, this could readily be achieved by a broadening of the remit of the existing Farm Animal Welfare Council.

One country already has such a committee: the Danish Ethical Council Concerning Animals. It is striking that the Danish committee is under the responsibility of their Ministry of Justice, whereas committees with similar but not identical remits in Belgium, Germany, The Netherlands, Sweden and the UK come under their Ministries of Agriculture.[20]

What about consensus and accountability? Few existing committees have sufficient public input, public profile or public accountability. Banner pointed out that:

> It is, of course, important that such a committee should secure the widest measure of public support. To that end it is essential that in its composition the committee should not only reflect the plurality of moral outlooks in our society, but that it should also be a forum for the rigorous development and examination of conflicting viewpoints.[18]

Similarly, Bernard Rollin has long argued for such a national committee in the USA, with a major element of public involvement.[21]

At the least, it is essential for public confidence in the safeguarding of animal welfare that the procedures of such committees should be well publicized. But why should we settle for the least option? Animal welfare is a topic that concerns the large majority of the public, and the public should have the opportunity to be involved in decisions that affect it. This could be achieved by public representation on committees, or by committees setting up consensus conferences to help them to make decisions. Either way, accountability would result.

It is salutary to realize that it is over 30 years since Ruth Harrison's book *Animal Machines*[22] raised public concern for animal welfare. The time is right for that concern to be responsibly addressed. If the public and welfare organizations will unite in pressing for establishment of animal welfare ethical advisory committees, and for other more specific changes where appropriate, it is achievable.

Such measures will not produce an ideal world for all animals. That is not possible. They will produce a compromise, but a compromise shifted further than hitherto in favour of animals. Animals help us and we should help them. Whether we concentrate on our duties or on the consequences of our actions, and whether we emphasize animal minds, bodies or natures, achieving a better compromise for animals is a priority for the opening years of the twenty-first century.

Conclusions

- While individual actions are important (Chapter 8), action on animal welfare must also be taken at the level of societies, by legislation, by creation of Codes of Practice and by international communication and negotiation.
- Pressures for 'free trade' and conformity of legislation between countries are slowing progress on welfare, particularly of farm animals. Ways to overcome this effect must be found, for example use of public subsidies for welfare improvements. Trade can also have positive effects on welfare, especially when companies such as supermarkets develop ethical policies based on the attitudes of their customers.
- Communication about animal welfare is vital. Attitudes are diverse, so it is important for people to attempt to understand each other's viewpoints. This should enable common principles to be established and practical measures to be taken that enable more co-operation in attempts to improve both human and animal welfare.
- The main conclusion of this book is that animal welfare ethical advisory committees should be established by national governments, with international communication and collaboration being expected and encouraged. These committees should have public input and accountability. If the public and welfare organizations increase pressure for such a change it

can be achieved, with the potential of making improvements in animal welfare that are long overdue.

References

1. Stevenson, P. (1996) This cynical trade must stop. *Agscene (The Quarterly Magazine of Compassion in World Farming)*, Autumn, 8–9.
2. Herscovici, A. (1985) *Second Nature: The Animal Rights Controversy.* CBC Enterprises, Toronto.
3. Care for the Wild/European Federation for Nature and Animals (1994) *Trapping Animals for Fur.* Care for the Wild, West Sussex.
4. McCrindle, C. (1998) The community development approach to animal welfare: an African perspective. *Applied Animal Behaviour Science*, **59**, 227–33.
5. Jorêt, A.D. (1998) Walking the animal welfare tight-rope – an egg industry view. In *Farm Animal Welfare: Who Writes the Rules? Programme & Summaries* (ed. British Society for Animal Science), p. 2. British Society for Animal Science, Edinburgh.
6. Ministry of Agriculture, Fisheries and Food (1987) *Codes of Recommendation for the Welfare of Livestock: Domestic Fowls.* Her Majesty's Stationery Office, London.
7. Holloway, I. (1998) *Public attitudes towards pig welfare in the UK.* MSc thesis, University of Edinburgh.
8. Bennett, R.M. (1997) Economics. In *Animal Welfare* (eds M.C. Appleby & B.O. Hughes), pp. 235–248. CAB International, Wallingford, UK.
9. Ministry of Agriculture, Fisheries and Food (1997) News release, 18th June.
10. Webster, A.J.F. (1994) *Animal Welfare: A Cool Eye Towards Eden.* Blackwell, Oxford.
11. RSPCA (undated) *Freedom Food leaflet.* Freedom Foods Ltd, West Sussex, UK.
12. Lowman, B. (1998) The producer's view: ruminants. In *Farm Animal Welfare: Who Writes the Rules? Programme & Summaries* (ed. British Society for Animal Science), p. 4. British Society for Animal Science, Edinburgh.
13. Watkins, K. (1998) Green trade dream that can turn turtle. *Guardian Weekly*, 4th October, p. 29.
14. The Humane Society of the United States (1998) *National Farm Animal Awareness Week leaflet.* The Humane Society of the United States, Washington DC.
15. Association for Study of Animal Behaviour videos *Let's Ask the Animals* and *Stimulus Response*, available from ASAB Membership Secretary, 82A High St, Sawston, Cambridge CB2 4HJ, UK.
16. UFAW (1999) *The UFAW Handbook on the Management and Welfare of*

Farm Animals, 4th edn (eds R. Ewbank & C.B. Hart). Universities Federation for Animal Welfare, Potters Bar, UK; UFAW (1999) *The UFAW Handbook on the Care and Management of Laboratory Animals*, 7th edn (ed. T.B. Poole). Blackwell Science, Oxford.

17. Lloyd-Evans, L.P.M. (1995) Representation of the people? The UK's first Consensus Conference. *Science and Engineering Ethics*, 1, 93–6.
18. Banner Committee (1995) *Report of the Committee to Consider the Ethical Implications of Emerging Technologies in the Breeding of Farm Animals.* Her Majesty's Stationery Office, London.
19. Coghlan, A. (1995) Altered animals need watchdog to protect them. *New Scientist*, 11th March, p. 12.
20. Spedding, C.R.W. (1996) *Agriculture and the Citizen.* Chapman and Hall, London.
21. Rollin, B.E. (1986) 'The Frankenstein Thing': the moral impact of genetic engineering of agricultural animals on society and future science. In *The Genetic Engineering of Agricultural Animals* (eds J.W. Evans & A. Hollaender), pp. 285–97. Plenum, New York; Rollin, B.E. (1995) *The Frankenstein Syndrome: Ethical and Social Issues in the Genetic Engineering of Animals.* Cambridge University Press, Cambridge.
22. Harrison, R. (1964) *Animal Machines: The New Factory Farming Industry.* Vincent Stuart, London.

Appendix – Some Useful Addresses

While a comprehensive list of sources is not possible here, the following selection may be of help and many will lead on to others in turn.

American Association for Laboratory Animal Science (AALAS)
70 Timber Creek Drive, Suite 5, Cordova, TN 38018, USA
http://www.aalas.org/

Animal Behavior Society (USA)
ABS Main Office: American Editorial Office for Animal Behaviour
2611 East 10th Street, #170, Indiana University, Bloomington, IN 47408-2603, USA
http://www.cisab.indiana.edu/ABS/index.html

Association for Study of Animal Behaviour
http://www.hbuk.co.uk/ap/asab

British Laboratory Animal Veterinary Association
c/o British Veterinary Association, 7 Mansfield Road, London W1M 0AT, UK

Compassion in World Farming
5A Charles Street, Petersfield, Hants GU32 3EH, UK

European Biomedical Research Association
58 Great Marlborough Street, London W1V 1DD, UK

European Centre for the Validation of Alternative Methods (ECVAM)
http://www.ei.jrc.it/report/ecvam.html

Fund for the Replacement of Animals in Medical Experimentation (FRAME)
Russell & Burch House, 9698 North Sherwood Street, Nottingham NG1 4EE, UK

Greenpeace (London)
Canonbury Villas, London N1 2PN, UK
http://www.greenpeace.org.uk/greenpeace.html

Health & Safety Executive (HSE)
Broad Lane, Sheffield S3 7HQ, UK
http://www.hse.gov.uk

Human–Animal Interactions Organisations
http://www.soton.ac.uk/~tobe/AzI/HAI_orgs.html

Humane Society and Animal Welfare Ring Homepage
http://incolor.inetnebr.com/acg/humane.html

Insitute of Laboratory Animal Resources (ILAR)
2101 Constitution Avenue, NW, Washington DC 20418, USA
http://www2.nas.edu/ilarhome/

Institute of Animal Technology
5 South Parade, Summertown, Oxford OX2 7JL, UK

International Society for Applied Ethology
http://www.sh.plym.ac.uk/isae/tsthome2.htm

Laboratory Animal Science Association
PO Box 3993, Tamworth, Staffs B78 3QU, UK

Laboratory Animals Ltd
c/o Royal Society of Medicine Press Ltd, 1 Wimpole Street, London W1M 8AE, UK

Ministry of Agriculture, Fisheries & Food (MAFF)
Hook Rise South, Tolworth, Surbiton, Surrey KT6 7NF, UK
http://www.maff.org.uk

National Farmers' Union (UK)
NFU, 164 Shaftesbury Avenue, London WC2H 8HL, UK
http://www.nfu.org.uk/

Netherlands Centre for Alternatives to Animal Use (NCA)
The Netherlands Centre, Alternatives to Animal Use (NCA), Yalelaan 17, NL-3584
CL UTRECHT, The Netherlands
http://www.pdk.dgk.ruu.nl/nca/nb3.htm

Norwegian School of Veterinary Science
P.O. Box 8146 Dep., N-0033 Oslo, Norway
http://oslovet.veths.no/NORINA/default.html

Research Animal Liaison Council
PO Box 2JD, London W1A 2JD, UK

Research Defence Society
58 Great Marlborough Street, London W1V 1DD, UK
http://www.uel.ac.ek:80/research/rds

Royal College of Veterinary Surgeons
Belgravia House, 6264 Horseferry Road, London SW1P 2AF, UK

Royal Society for the Prevention of Cruelty to Animals (RSPCA)
Enquiries Service, RSPCA, The Causeway, Horsham, West Sussex RH12 1HG, UK
http://www.rspca.org.uk

University of California Center for Animal Alternatives
School of Veterinary Medicine, University of California, Davis, USA
http://www.vetmed.ucdavis.edu/Animal_Alternatives/organiza.htm

Universities Federation for Animal Welfare (UFAW)
The Old School, Brewhouse Hill, Wheathampstead, Herts AL4 8AN, UK
http://www.users.dircon.co.uk/~ufaw3/

USDA Animal Welfare Information Center
The Animal Welfare Information Center, U.S. Department of Agriculture,
Agricultural Research Service, National Agricultural Library 10301 Baltimore
Avenue, 5th Floor, Beltsville, MD 20705-2351, USA
http://www.nal.usda.gov/awic/

Index